Smoking Cessation Matters in Primary Care

Marcus Munafò

Mark Drury

Gill Wakley

and

Ruth Chambers

with

Mike Murphy

RADCLIFFE MEDICAL PRESS

Radcliffe Medical Press Ltd
18 Marcham Road
Abingdon
Oxon OX14 1AA
United Kingdom

www.radcliffe-oxford.com
The Radcliffe Medical Press electronic catalogue and online ordering facility.
Direct sales to anywhere in the world.

British Library Cataloguing in Publication Data

A catalogue record for this book is available from the British Library.

ISBN 1 85775 442 5

Typeset by Joshua Associates Ltd, Oxford
Printed and bound by TJ International Ltd, Padstow, Cornwall

Contents

Preface

The material in this book sets out how learning more about smoking and smoking-related conditions can be incorporated into your personal development plan. You need to develop a dual focus on improving the management of smoking and related issues, and increasing the efficiency of the working environment in primary care. Practice team members should work together to direct their individual learning plans to form their practice personal and professional development plan. This should complement the business plan of the practice or primary care group/trust in England, the local health group in Wales or their equivalent bodies in the rest of the UK (all termed primary care organisations (PCOs) hereafter).

You may decide to allocate 50% of the time you intend to spend drawing up and applying a personal development plan in any one year to learning more about smoking. You might include smoking cessation in the more general area of health promotion, or in related conditions such as the management of coronary heart disease. That would leave space in your learning plan for other important topics such as mental health or cancer – whatever is a priority for you, your practice team and your patient population. There will be some overlap between topics. For example, you cannot consider a person who smokes in isolation from their other lifestyle risk factors, and that means understanding and knowing how to prevent and manage cardiovascular problems, too.

Chapter 8 of the book describes how a clinical governance culture incorporates effective clinical management and well-organised working conditions. You should be able to demonstrate that you are fit to practise as an individual clinician or manager (best practice in the management of smoking in this case) and that your working environment is fit to practise from. This section will be relevant to all readers, whether you are a clinician or a primary care manager, as it will enable you to understand more of the context within which you work and how your individual contribution fits into the whole picture of healthcare.

Each chapter gradually builds up your knowledge base of smoking so that you can bring yourself up to date with the most recent evidence. There have been a great many changes in recommended best practice in the last few years, as major research has provided evidence for effective interventions.

The whole programme builds up to the composing of a personal development plan and a practice personal and professional development plan in Chapters 9 and 10. Interactive exercises at the end of each chapter give the reader an opportunity to assess their learning needs, review their performance or that of the practice organisation, and reflect on what improvements to make.

You should transfer information from these needs assessment exercises to the relevant slots in your personal development plan as an individual, or your practice personal and professional development plan if you are working as a team. Adopt a wide-based approach to improving quality – think of how you are establishing a clinical governance culture in your own practice team through your timed action plans.

What should you do next?

Study the templates for a personal development plan or a practice personal and professional development plan (also termed a 'practice learning plan') on pages 169–178 and 193–199. You will be filling these in as you go along. Decide whether you will be starting out on your personal development plan or working with colleagues on the practice learning plan. Everyone's personal development plans should mesh with the practice learning plan by the time they have finished drawing them up.

Make changes as a result – to your workplace, or to the equipment in your practice, or to the advice you give patients, or to the way in which you manage smoking or complicating clinical problems associated with it.

Marcus Munafò
November 2002

About the authors

Marcus Munafò is a psychologist and Research Fellow for the Cancer Research UK GP Research Group, based at Oxford University. His particular area of interest is the neurobiology of nicotine addiction, with a view to developing novel smoking-cessation interventions, and tailoring existing interventions to individuals. In particular, his research focuses on the role of changes in reward pathways following repeated use of nicotine, and the behavioural changes that occur as a consequence of this.

His teaching responsibilities are mainly in the Department of Experimental Psychology and on the Oxford Clinical Course, and he also advised on the setting up of the Oxfordshire Smoking Cessation Service. Marcus is a lecturer on the MRCPsych Part I Wessex Course, and he lectures widely on addiction in general and nicotine addiction in particular, and has provided consultancy services on these topics to pharmaceutical companies.

Mark Drury is a general practitioner in Oxfordshire, a Macmillan Cancer Lead for his PCO and a Research Fellow for the Cancer Research UK GP Research Group at Oxford University, where the focus of research is the treatment and consequences of nicotine addiction.

Mark entered general practice sufficiently long ago to be able to recall that filling a pipe with tobacco during the surgery coffee break did not raise eyebrows. His subsequent 20 years in general practice have given him clinical experience in smoking cessation work, an insight into the organisational aspects of setting up practice-based services for smokers, and a feeling of wistful nostalgia for the perfume of ready rubbed tobacco.

In the wider field of cancer he has an interest in shared care, and he has published studies on patient-held records, reported on shared cancer care in Europe, and written about aspects of clinical management in palliative care.

His more eclectic work has included publications on the history of general practice in the NHS, and on clinical negligence, and he has a continuing interest in patient participation in primary care.

Ruth Chambers has been a GP for 20 years and is currently Professor of Primary Care Development at Staffordshire University. She holds several national posts such as the Lead for Education for the NHS Alliance, and National Convenor of the Royal College of General Practitioners' Accredited Professional Development (APD) programme, and she is a member of the Children's Taskforce for England.

Ruth has designed and organised many types of educational initiatives, including distance-learning programmes. Recently she has developed a keen interest in working with GPs, nurses and others in primary care around clinical governance and practice personal and professional development plans. She and Gill Wakley have produced a new series of books designed to help readers to draw up their own personal development plans or practice learning plans around important clinical topics, such as diabetes.

Gill Wakley started in general practice in 1966, but transferred to community medicine shortly afterwards and then into public health. A desire for increased contact with patients caused a move back into general practice, together with community gynaecology, in 1978. She has been combining the two, in varying amounts, ever since. Throughout she has been heavily involved in learning and teaching. She was in a training general practice, became an instructing doctor and a regional assessor in family planning, and was until recently a Senior Clinical Lecturer in the Primary Care Department at Keele University. Like Ruth, she has run all types of educational initiatives and activities, from individual mentoring and instruction to small-group work, plenary lectures, distance-learning programmes, workshops and courses for a wide range of health professionals and lay people.

She briefly worked for Quit (the UK charity that offers help to people who want to stop smoking), and she continues to encourage people to tackle this important public health problem.

Mike Murphy practised medicine for several years, latterly in general practice, but he left clinical work for a career in research many years ago. He has directed the Cancer Research UK GP Research Group in the Department of Primary Health Care at the University of Oxford since 1997. The research group's main interests are cancer prevention and in particular smoking. The study of the different disciplines that contribute to the 'science of smoking cessation' is now his main concern, overshadowing previously established interests in the role of endogenous hormones in the development of breast and gynaecological cancers.

He is fascinated by, but has much to learn about, psychology, pharmacology, neuroscience and molecular genetics, which he believes will contribute to a better understanding of how to help smokers to give up with help from primary care, and will thus make a big difference to the public's health.

CHAPTER 1

Smoking initiation, nicotine addiction and the smoking life-course

> It is the only product which kills people when used *as intended*.

More than a quarter of adults in the UK smoke 15 cigarettes a day or more, while approximately 15% of children aged between 11 and 15 years smoke once a week or more. However, the majority (around 70%) of adult smokers are keen to stop, and one-third of smokers make at least one attempt to stop in any given year. Yet only 2% of smokers successfully stop smoking every year. In the UK, 80% of those who become regular smokers do so by the age of 18 years, and 90% by the age of 19 years. There are currently approximately 10 million smokers in the UK, and somewhat more who have given up without pharmacotherapy. The possibility therefore exists that those who remain are, on average, more addicted. The history of smoking cessation is a long one, with anti-smoking campaigns being reported as far back as the seventeenth and eighteenth centuries. However, only recently has it become generally accepted that nicotine is the principal addictive component of tobacco and that, because of this, smoking initiation will in many cases result in addiction.

History of tobacco use

Introduction of nicotine

The use of tobacco as a psychoactive substance began in the Americas, possibly as early as 6000 BC, and was introduced to Europe almost immediately after Columbus's voyages. The practice was introduced into English society in 1565, although it did not become widely popular until about 20 years later. The methods of delivery used by Native Americans included smoking, snuffing and drinking of various tobacco preparations. The use of tobacco was associated with medical and religious rituals, and a ban on the use of tobacco was included in a Papal decree of 1586, although this was motivated by a desire to prevent the contamination of Christian rituals by Native American religious rituals, rather than being a result of any health considerations. Indeed, the early growth in popularity of tobacco was a consequence of its supposed healing properties, and it was widely regarded as a medicinal plant. It was not until the beginning of the seventeenth century that the supposed benefits of smoking tobacco began to be questioned, notably by King James I in his 'Counterblaste to Tobacco':

> a custome lothsome to the eye, hateful to the Nose, hermful to the braine, dangerous to the Lungs, and in the blacke stinking fume therof, nearest resembling the horrible Stigian smoke of the pit that is bottomlesse.

This concern continued into the eighteenth century, with an increasing number of physicians warning of the potential dangers of tobacco consumption, including its association with cancers of the nose (in the case of snuff takers) and of the lip (in the case of pipe smokers).

Patterns of tobacco consumption in Europe changed from its introduction in the sixteenth century, when the delivery device of choice was the pipe, through the eighteenth century, when snuff was commonly used, to the nineteenth century, when snuff-taking declined and cigar smoking became popular. It was not until the twentieth century that cigarette smoking became the most common form of tobacco consumption, some 50 years after the invention of this delivery device. The invention of the manufactured (as opposed to hand-prepared) cigarette led to the habit of tobacco smoking being adopted by the majority of the population, to the extent that cigarettes were included as part of the daily rations issued to soldiers in the First World War. The prevalence of tobacco smoking in the UK reached 70% in men and 50% in women between the 1940s and the 1960s, and then declined in the early 1970s as increasing evidence of the health consequences of tobacco use became available.

The rise of the cigarette

The cigarette, although apparently so simple in construction, is in fact a highly efficient delivery device for tobacco and nicotine, and is a highly

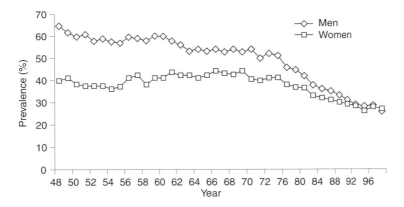

Figure 1.1: Prevalence of smoking of manufactured cigarettes in men and women in Great Britain, 1948–1997.
Source: 1948–71 Tobacco Advisory Council data, 1972–96 General Household Survey and 1997 Omnibus Survey.

engineered product. The Freedom of Information Act in the USA has resulted in revealing insights into the mind of tobacco manufacturers:

> The cigarette should be conceived not as a product but as a package. The product is nicotine. Think of the cigarette pack as a storage container for a day's supply of nicotine ... Think of the cigarette as the dispenser for a dose unit of nicotine ... Smoke is beyond question the most optimised vehicle of nicotine and the cigarette the most optimised dispenser of smoke.[1]

A cigarette consists primarily of a paper tube that contains chopped tobacco leaf and 'filler' (stems and other parts of the tobacco plant that are essentially waste, although they do contain nicotine), and a filter made of cellulose acetate. An increase in the filler content reduces the density of tobacco leaf and results in a lower tar delivery, and this varies across brands. The type of paper that is used can influence how much air is drawn into the cigarette, thereby diluting the smoke. The filter traps some of the particulate content of cigarette smoke and cools the smoke, making it easier to inhale.

In addition to the physical construction of the cigarette, the chemical engineering of the content contributes to its effectiveness. In the manufacture of cigarettes a large number of additives are permissible, including humectants to prolong shelf-life, sugars to make the smoke milder and therefore easier to inhale, and flavourings to improve the taste of the smoke. Another group of additives that are commonly used are ammonia compounds, which raise the alkalinity of cigarette smoke, thereby increasing the concentration of unbound nicotine in cigarette smoke and in turn increasing the speed with which nicotine is absorbed. In total around 600 additives are permitted, contributing to around 10% of the cigarette by weight. In practice, the actual number of additives used in the manufacture of different brands, and their exact function, are often unknown.

In the 1970s, various changes in the manufacture of cigarettes were introduced by voluntary agreement between governments and the tobacco industry in response to growing concern about the health effects of cigarette smoking, in particular in relation to lung cancer. These changes led to the introduction of 'low-tar' cigarettes, which resulted in lower tar yields in the particulate phase of cigarette smoke (e.g. by using filters that drew in more air, thereby diluting the smoke). In 1970, tar yields were typically 20 mg per cigarette, whereas a limit of 12 mg per cigarette was set by the European Union to be achieved by 1997. This will be replaced by a new directive requiring all cigarettes sold within the European Union to conform to a maximum tar yield of 10 mg per cigarette and a maximum nicotine yield of 1 mg per cigarette. However, these figures for tar yield (and corresponding nicotine yield) are generated from data on machine-smoked cigarettes, and there is increasing evidence that these data are of little relevance to nicotine and tar yields in cigarettes smoked by humans, since smoking behaviour can be modified to achieve the desired intake. For example, tar and nicotine yields can be increased by puffing on a cigarette more often, by inhaling more deeply or by blocking the filter holes with one's fingers. Such compensatory behaviour suggests that the health benefits of changing to low-tar cigarettes may be lower than anticipated. This view is supported by recent evidence which shows that the nicotine and tar yields from machine-smoked cigarettes are poor predictors of nicotine intake (and therefore tar intake, since the two are highly correlated) in smokers.[2]

Cigarette smoking in the UK

The vast majority of tobacco users in the UK are cigarette smokers (approximately 10 million adults, compared with around 2 million cigar and/or pipe users). There are also a similar number of ex-smokers. The highest prevalence of cigarette smoking, when surveys were first conducted, was in 1948, when the prevalence among men was 82%. In women the figure was lower, and it gradually rose to a peak of 45% in the mid-1960s. The prevalence of cigarette smoking then declined as the health risks became more widely known, and it fell faster in men than in women, so that there is now no significant difference between men and women as a whole. However, there are signs that this decline

Table 1.1 Prevalence of cigarette smoking by age in the UK (1998)

Age (years)	1996	1998
16–19	29%	31%
20–24	39%	40%
25–34	37%	35%
35–49	30%	30%
50–59	27%	27%
≥60	18%	16%

Source: Centre for Public Health Monitoring.[3]

has begun to tail off, and there is also evidence of an increase in prevalence among certain age groups.

Cigarette smoking is also more common among those employed in manual occupations compared with those employed in non-manual occupations, partly due to a slower decline in cigarette smoking in the former group.

There are also regional differences in the prevalence of smoking. For example, 22% of the population of East Anglia smoke compared with 31% of the population of North-West England.

In 1999–2000, the Government received £7600 million in revenue on the sale of cigarettes, in the form of duty and VAT. Approximately 80% of the retail price of a packet of cigarettes consists of tax in one of these two forms, and increasing taxation has been the principal means by which the tobacco policy of successive governments has been implemented. There is evidence that this has a modest effect on cigarette consumption and also results in some smokers stopping the habit. The net effect over time has been an increase in the average price per pack that has outstripped the rate of inflation to a considerable degree.

Table 1.2 Prevalence of cigarette smoking by socio-economic group (1999)

	Professional	Employers and managers	Intermediate non-manual	Skilled manual	Semi-skilled manual	Unskilled manual
Men	13%	20%	23%	34%	39%	44%
Women	14%	24%	23%	28%	34%	33%

Source: Action on Smoking and Health.[4]

Pharmacology of nicotine

Absorption

Tobacco smoke consists of both volatile and particulate phases. The volatile phase includes several hundred gaseous compounds (e.g. carbon monoxide), while the particulate phase is composed of several thousand compounds, the most significant of which is the alkaloid nicotine. Absorption of nicotine from burning tobacco is dependent on the pH of the smoke. This in turn depends on the method used for curing the tobacco. For example, smoke from cigar and pipe tobacco is alkaline and is readily absorbed in the mouth, but it is also harsher and therefore less likely to be inhaled deeply. However, smoke from cigarette tobacco is more acidic and must be inhaled into the lungs to be absorbed effectively. It is also less harsh, partly due to the presence of additives that are introduced during the curing process. Menthol cigarettes allow deeper inhalation because they are less harsh, which results in a risk of adenocarcinoma of the peripheral lung rather than squamous-cell carcinoma of the bronchus. The nicotine in cigarette smoke is therefore inhaled and deposited in the airways and alveoli. It is then rapidly absorbed into systemic arterial blood, and it reaches the brain within 10–20 seconds. Levels of nicotine in arterial blood can be up to six times those found in venous blood. This is relevant to an understanding of the addictive properties of nicotine from cigarette smoke, because while venous blood levels of nicotine after smoking a single cigarette peak after around 10 minutes and then gradually decline, the concentration of nicotine in arterial blood peaks and drops sharply after each inhalation. This strengthens the reinforcing (i.e. addictive) properties of nicotine that is absorbed in this way.

Nicotine from oral products such as chewing tobacco and nasal products such as snuff is absorbed through the mucosa, and nicotine levels rise more slowly when these products are used than in cigarette smoking. The different rates of absorption when such products are used mean that the behavioural reinforcement offered by these delivery devices is far less than that offered by cigarettes. In addition, the rapid delivery of nicotine offered by cigarette smoking allows fine titration of the plasma nicotine level in order to achieve the desired effect.

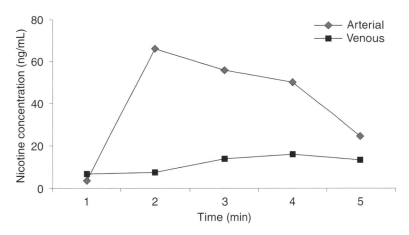

Figure 1.2: Time-course of arterial and venous nicotine concentrations. *Source*: Henningfield *et al.* (1993).[5]

Mechanisms of action

Recent animal and cellular physiology studies have provided substantial insight into the mechanisms of action of nicotine in the brain. In particular, the areas of the brain, the types of receptor and the changes in neuronal activity that mediate the effects of nicotine use have been described in some detail. Nicotinic acetylcholine receptors are found distributed throughout the brain, being concentrated in the cortex and thalamus, but also found in significant concentrations in the amygdala, septum, brainstem and locus coereleus. The direct activation of these nicotinic receptor sites mediates the effects of nicotine consumption. Of particular interest for understanding the mechanisms of nicotine addiction is the high level of expression of nicotinic receptors in brain areas associated with learning and reinforcement, such as the mesolimbic system.

Addictive substances such as nicotine are positively reinforcing as a consequence of their ability to enhance neurotransmission along dopaminergic pathways in the mesolimbic system, in particular the nucleus accumbens. In animal studies, lesions to the mesolimbic system substantially reduce the ability of addictive substances to act as positive reinforcers in a self-administration paradigm. This system therefore almost certainly constitutes at least a part of the common pathway that underlies the mechanism of all addictive substances in humans.

Individual differences in nicotine metabolism and sensitivity to nicotine

Pharmacokinetics and metabolism

Nicotine is metabolised extensively in the liver, and to a lesser extent in the lungs and kidneys. The half-life of nicotine is approximately two hours. The level of nicotine following administration depends on the balance of the rate of intake and the rate of elimination, both of which are subject to considerable inter-individual differences in the case of nicotine. The primary metabolite of nicotine is cotinine (70%), which has a substantially longer half-life (averaging around 16 hours) than nicotine, and is therefore often used as a validator of smoking status over the previous 2–3 days and as a biochemical marker of nicotine consumption. Exhaled carbon monoxide has a shorter half-life, and is used to validate smoking status over the previous 12–18 hours, with a cut-off value of 10 parts per million generally being used to indicate no smoking over that period. Serum thiocyanate levels can also be used to validate smoking status.

Systematic sex differences in nicotine metabolism have also been reported, such that the clearance of nicotine appears to be greater in men than in women. However, this does *not* mean that the level of nicotine in the blood is necessarily substantially different across individuals, or across men and women. Instead, it appears that nicotine administration is titrated so as to maintain a consistent blood nicotine concentration. For example, it has been found that men smoke cigarettes more frequently than women, with the result that total blood nicotine levels in both groups are similar. There are also substantial intra-individual differences in nicotine absorption, which are exacerbated by the choice of delivery device (e.g. cigarette) and differences in the use of the delivery device (i.e. pattern of smoking behaviour). For example, cigarettes deliver their nicotine content to the brain within approximately 10 seconds, whereas nicotine levels rise far more slowly when oral or nasal tobacco products, such as chewing tobacco or snuff, are used.

Effects on human performance

The popularity of nicotine as a social drug suggests that this compound, especially as delivered by cigarette smoke, offers at least

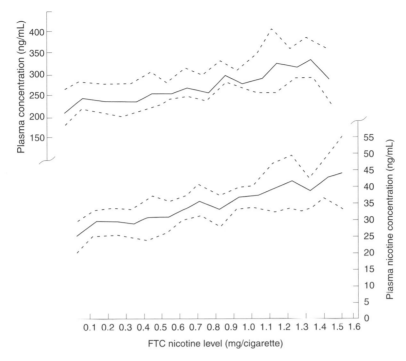

Figure 1.3: Plasma cotinine and nicotine concentrations in cigarette smokers according to the FTC nicotine yield. Solid lines indicate mean; broken lines indicate 95% confidence intervals.
Source: Gori and Lynch (1985).[6]

some attractive benefits and effects on performance, mood, etc. which may contribute to the addictive properties of nicotine. Anecdotal and subjective evidence would certainly suggest that arousal control, mood control, improved concentration and anxiety control are some of the consequences of nicotine consumption that lead to its repeated administration. Interestingly, the results from laboratory studies that have investigated these effects have been more equivocal, particularly with regard to the role of nicotine in controlling negative affect and stress. In this case, the evidence appears to suggest that it is nicotine deprivation that results in elevated anxiety and vulnerability to stress, the effects of which can be ameliorated by the administration of nicotine. Negative affect is therefore a withdrawal effect of nicotine, such that nicotine administration does not in itself reduce negative affect that has arisen for other reasons.

However, in the case of other aspects of behaviour there is evidence that performance benefits resulting from the administration of nicotine are not a consequence of the relief of withdrawal deficits. Visual

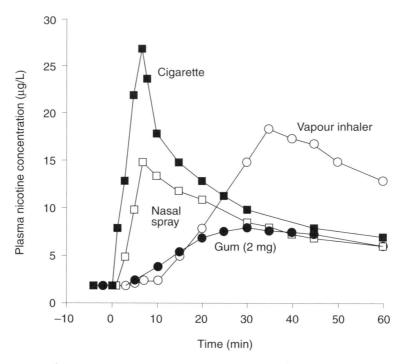

Figure 1.4: Plasma nicotine concentrations during and after drug administration, shown for four different nicotine delivery systems.
Source: Modified from Schneider NG (1992) Nicotine therapy in smoking cessation: pharmacokinetic considerations. *Clin Pharmacokin.* **23**: 169–72.

perception, motor function and cognitive performance all appear to be facilitated, in absolute terms, by the administration of nicotine, even in the case of regular smokers. Importantly, these effects are a specific consequence of the nicotine content of cigarette smoke, and they may be positively reinforcing in themselves.

Addictive substances generally exhibit two common characteristics. First, they act as positive reinforcers, in both self-administration paradigms in animals and in human studies, and secondly, following chronic exposure, tolerance of the drug results in the use of increasing doses and the withdrawal of the substance elicits a range of symptoms, the effects of which can be ameliorated by resumption of administration of the substance. In the case of nicotine, common withdrawal symptoms include the following:

- increased irritation/aggression
- increased negative affect/anxiety
- cravings for tobacco
- increased appetite
- mouth ulcers.

Smoking initiation in early to mid-adolescence

Personality and smoking initiation

The concept of an addictive personality is well established in the popular imagination, but evidence for the existence of a single personality dimension or type associated with addictive behaviours is minimal. Nevertheless, certain personality dimensions drawn from personality trait theory have been reliably shown to be associated with aspects of addictive behaviours in general, and smoking behaviours in particular. However, studies designed to investigate the association between personality dimensions and smoking behaviour have been hindered by the range of personality measures that exist, many of which overlap in their conceptual and theoretical scope. Moreover, although personality differences between groups of smokers and non-smokers have been reliably demonstrated, this does not provide much insight into the causal basis of such an association.

Two broad models of personality exist. Five-factor models assume that behaviours are broadly consistent and can be *described* along five dimensions, but that these dimensions reflect nothing more than behavioural consistency. Three-factor models, on the other hand, assume that individual differences in behaviour can be mapped along three dimensions that reflect underlying individual differences in brain function. Arguably such models provide a firmer basis for understanding the causal mechanisms underlying any association between personality and smoking behaviour. However, these two approaches are not incompatible, and although various questionnaire measures of personality use different names to describe the dimensions of personality, there is a growing consensus regarding the handful of traits along which human behaviour can be reliably shown to vary.

The most consistently reported association between smoking behaviour and personality relates to the personality dimension of sensation seeking (also variously described as novelty seeking, experience seeking, etc.) in five-factor models, and extraversion (which shares a substantial function overlap with the former dimension) and neuroticism in three-factor models. For example, extraversion has been explained as being a function of low cortical arousal, resulting in behaviours that lead to an increase in such arousal. This hypothesis would predict a positive association between high levels of extraversion and smoking behaviour, and there is some evidence to support this relationship. The evidence for a positive association between neuroticism and smoking behaviour is more equivocal, but there is some evidence that smokers who smoke in order to control negative affect report higher levels of neuroticism. Alternative models of personality are based on individual differences in sensitivity to reward and punishment. Sensitivity to reward is conceptually closely related to the extraversion and neuroticism dimensions of three-factor models (and may be calculated from scores on questionnaire measures of these two dimensions) and the novelty-seeking dimension of five-factor models. This suggests that smoking initiation may be associated with sensitivity to reward. That is, individuals who score high on measures of the sensitivity to reward dimension might be more likely to smoke because the reinforcing properties of nicotine exert a proportionately greater effect than its aversive properties.

The personality traits that have been reported to be associated with smoking behaviour appear to be highly heritable (i.e. they have an important genetic contribution), and there is increasing support for the notion that the genetic influence on smoking initiation is mediated by personality. For example, there is evidence for a positive association between certain personality traits and specific polymorphisms (e.g. novelty-seeking behaviour and polymorphisms in dopamine D4 receptors). Moreover, the association between personality and smoking behaviour has been reported in populations where smoking is still regarded as socially acceptable, undermining the suggestion that the relationship between personality and smoking behaviour is a function of rebellious behaviour that is better represented at the extremes of certain personality dimensions. Inherited differences in sensitivity to reward or to punishment, which may also be described along other overlapping personality dimensions, may represent an important risk factor for smoking initiation (and possibly for initiation of any potentially addictive behaviour). Such shared risk factors for addictive behaviours that are not unique to nicotine addiction may interact with inherited individual differences that are unique to nicotine addiction, such as nicotine metabolism, which may enhance or diminish the reinforcing properties of nicotine.

Family and peer influences

Risk factors for smoking are varied, and making inferences about the causal basis of such associations is hazardous. The factor most clearly associated with smoking behaviour is socio-economic status, with smoking prevalence being lowest in professional occupational groups and highest in semi-skilled manual occupational groups. Indeed, although smoking prevalence has declined markedly in the population as a whole over the last 20 years, this is largely due to a very substantial decline in prevalence in professional occupational groups. In the most deprived socio-economic groups, the prevalence of smoking has remained relatively unchanged and cessation rates have not increased. The difference between manual and non-manual groups has therefore widened, this gap being most marked in women. There is also regional variation, which is likely to be largely due to systematic differences in the socio-economic demographics of different regions. The lowest prevalence of smoking in adults is in the South and West NHS Region, and the highest prevalence is in the North-West NHS Region.

Given the addictive potential of nicotine, smoking initiation is an important concern, since prevention of this will prevent the subsequent development of a smoking habit. Risk factors for smoking initiation in children (i.e. those aged between 11 and 15 years) include the following:

- low educational attainment
- parents who are smokers
- siblings who are smokers
- peers/friends who are smokers
- teachers who are smokers.

One implication of this is that by reducing the overall prevalence of smoking, it should also be possible to reduce the risk of initiation in the population.

These factors are in addition to the broader predictors of smoking behaviour, such as socio-economic status. It has been suggested that children and adolescents smoke for different reasons to the majority of adult smokers, in that they smoke for the pleasurable consequences of nicotine administration, rather than to avoid the withdrawal effects of not smoking.

The media and advertising

It has been estimated that approximately £100 million is spent on advertising by the tobacco industry in the UK annually. The impact of this tobacco advertising on tobacco consumption has been the subject of substantial debate, resulting in official reviews in the USA, the UK and several other countries. The effect of tobacco advertising is made difficult to assess due to the range of methodologies used to answer the question, as well as the often poor quality of the data collected. The

Smee Report, published in the UK in 1992, concludes that in the case of advertising bans as a means of reducing smoking prevalence, 'the current evidence available . . . indicates a significant effect. In each case the banning of advertising was followed by a fall in smoking on a scale which cannot reasonably be attributed to other factors.'[7]

Other evidence cited in the Smee Report includes the association between advertising expenditure and overall consumption, and differences in consumption across countries with different levels of control over tobacco advertising. However, in each of these cases the evidence is less easy to interpret, as questions will always remain about the direction of causation. Nevertheless, taken together this body of evidence as presented in the Smee Report is highly suggestive of an association between advertising and smoking prevalence. The report does suggest that the effects of any advertising ban are likely to be modest, and a 2.5% reduction in consumption has been tentatively suggested. Moreover, this effect will not be immediately apparent, but will occur after a short period of time during which the residual effects of previous advertising disappear. Yet a figure of 2.5% should not be ignored, as it equates to between 1500 and 3000 lives a year that could be saved by such measures in the UK. This effect would be in addition to any reduction in the number of individuals taking up the smoking habit, which would obviously accrue benefits over a much longer period. It should be borne in mind that any money which is not spent by the consumer because of a reduction in cigarette sales is not lost to the economy, as it is likely to be spent on other goods and services. The argument that the money saved by the NHS on the care of those with smoking-related diseases as a result of reducing the number of smokers is in fact offset by the decrease in money gained through taxation of tobacco products is therefore false, as money which is not spent on tobacco products would most probably be spent on other (taxable) products.

At present, tobacco regulation in the UK includes both legal and voluntary controls, although the introduction of new legal measures (e.g. bans on tobacco advertising) means that the balance is continually shifting, in general in the direction of legal rather than voluntary controls. Relevant legal controls include the Children and Young Persons (Protection from Tobacco) Act 1991,[8] which strengthened existing laws on the sale of tobacco products to those under 16 years of age, and the Health and Safety at Work Act 1974,[9] which places restrictions on places (e.g. those where food is being prepared) as to where smoking is allowed. There has also been an increase in the numbers of employers and organisations that impose restrictions on smoking (e.g. the prohibition of smoking on transport services), and the majority of large companies in the UK now have a formal policy on smoking.

Genetic contribution to smoking initiation

Smoking behaviour and nicotine addiction have generated far less behavioural genetics research than other addictive behaviours, such as alcoholism. This is despite evidence from animal studies which suggests that key factors, such as the number and distribution of nicotinic receptors and the development of nicotine tolerance, are under a strong genetic influence. However, the evidence that does exist from twin, adoption and separated twin studies has consistently suggested that smoking behaviour has a strong genetic component. Heritability coefficients ranging from 0.28 to 0.85 for the risk of being a current smoker have been reported. Behavioural genetics studies allow the relative contribution of genetic, shared environmental and unique environmental influences to be distinguished, with the heritability coefficient itself reflecting the former. This means that between 28% and 85% of the observed variation in current smoking behaviour in the population from which the data were collected can be accounted for by genetic factors. Indeed, it has been suggested that the evidence for a genetic influence on smoking behaviour is stronger than the evidence for a genetic influence on alcoholism. Moreover, these studies have also indicated that these genetic factors relate to two distinct aspects of smoking behaviour, namely initiation and persistence.

Given the strong evidence for a genetic influence on current smoking status, the question of how this influence acts then arises. One possibility is that any genetic influence acts at the stage of smoking initiation, with subsequent smoking persistence being determined by environmental influences. Another possibility is that the reverse is true, and that smoking initiation is largely determined by environmental influences, while smoking persistence is influenced by genetic factors. Finally, there may be some combination of both, whereby a genetic influence exists for both smoking initiation and smoking persistence. In such a combined model some genetic influences might influence both initiation and persistence, while others might influence one or the other uniquely.

By comparing concordance rates for being a current smoker or an ex-smoker compared with never having smoked, the question of whether a genetic contribution to smoking initiation exists can be addressed. Such comparisons suggest that there is indeed such a contribution. For example, heritability coefficients of 0.44 in women and 0.51 in men for smoking initiation have been reported in a sample of Swedish adults born between 1926 and 1958.[10] It is also worth noting that a strong influence of shared environmental factors on smoking initiation and persistence is reported in this study, with little evidence of a role for unique environmental influences. The genetic risk factor for smoking initiation is reported elsewhere, and although the overall conclusion is robust, the specific heritability coefficients reported by individual studies are highly variable, ranging from below 0.30 to above 0.80. The role of shared environmental influences on initiation and persistence is also inconsistent across various populations, with some studies reporting minimal shared environmental influences. Sex differences in heritability coefficients are generally either not reported or minimal.

Taken together, these findings suggest that although there is consistent evidence for a genetic influence on smoking initiation, and substantial evidence for a shared environmental influence on initiation and persistence, the relative importance of genetic and environmental factors is highly variable across populations. For example, different heritability coefficients have been reported for smoking behaviour in African-Americans compared with white Americans.[10] Nevertheless, evidence from non-Western cultures suggests that the genetic influence on smoking behaviour remains an important risk factor even in populations where there are much higher rates of smoking (e.g. China). It is important to appreciate that reported heritability coefficients will vary with environmental factors, such as the prevalence of smoking. For example, some of the highest heritability coefficients for smoking initiation have been reported in studies on the Vietnam era twin population, where the participants were members of the US army at a time when smoking prevalence in the military services was very high. This natural experiment, where environmental variation in initiation is minimised, may account for the high heritability coefficients observed in this study.

Although an understanding of smoking initiation is clearly of importance for understanding the aetiology of nicotine addiction, it is smoking persistence that is responsible for the adverse health consequences of smoking. The evidence for a genetic influence on smoking persistence (studies comparing current smokers with ex-smokers) is also strong, with several studies reporting heritability coefficients above 0.50 for smoking persistence in both men and women. Interpretation of this result is complicated by the fact that the same genetic factors that influence smoking initiation could also influence persistence. Heath and Martin[11] have proposed three different models. The first is a 'single liability' model, in which the genetic and environmental influences are the same for smoking initiation and smoking persistence. The second is an 'independent liability' model, in which the factors that influence initiation and persistence are entirely independent. The third is a combined model in which some factors influence both initiation and persistence and other factors are unique to one or the other aspect of smoking behaviour. The third model has been reported to provide the best fit. In this model some ex-smokers are 'early quitters' who begin smoking but nevertheless have a low risk for initiation and do not continue their habit. Other ex-smokers are 'successful quitters' who begin smoking and continue their habit, but have a low risk for persistence and can therefore quit relatively easily. The balance of evidence suggests that whereas risk for smoking initiation is influenced by both genetic and environmental factors, risk of smoking persistence is primarily a function of genetic factors, with some of the genetic influence on smoking behaviour contributing to risk for both smoking initiation and persistence, as well as the amount smoked and the degree of dependence.

There is also evidence that some of the genetic influence on smoking persistence is not unique to smoking behaviour and is common to other addictions. For example, a degree of shared risk for nicotine dependence (as defined by DSM-III-R, in this case) and alcohol dependence has been reported. One suggestion is that this shared risk relates to predisposition to the development of facilitated neurotransmission in reward pathways that can then be activated by other addicting substances.

Reflection exercise

Exercise 1

How many people have you identified as smokers in your practice population? How do the proportions compare with the national figures given in this chapter? Do you need to redouble your efforts to identify smokers from among your patients and update their medical records?

Now that you have completed this interactive reflection exercise, transfer the information to the empty template of the personal development plan on pages 169–178 if you are working on your own learning plan, or to the practice personal and professional development plan on pages 193–199 if you are working on a practice team learning plan. Don't forget to keep the evidence of your learning in your personal portfolio.

References

1 Quote ascribed to William L Dunn Jr, Philip Morris, researcher, after attending a 1972 meeting held by the Council for Tobacco Research.
2 Jarvis MJ, Primatesta P, Boreham R and Feyerabend C (2001) Nicotine yield from machine-smoked cigarettes and nicotine intakes in smokers: evidence from a representative population survey. *J Natl Cancer Inst.* **93**: 134–8.
3 Centre for Public Health Monitoring (1999) *Compendium of Clinical and Health Indicators.* Centre for Public Health Monitoring, London.
4 Action on Smoking and Health (2002) http://www.ash.org.uk/.
5 Henningfield JE, Cohen C and Pickworth WB (1993) Psychopharmacology of nicotine. In: CT Orleans and JD Slade (eds) *Nicotine Addiction: principles and management.* Oxford University Press, New York.
6 Gori GB and Lynch CJ (1985) Analytical cigarette yields as predictors of smoke bioavailability. *Regul Toxicol Pharmacol.* **5**: 314–26.
7 SMEE Report, The (1992) *Effect of Tobacco Advertising on Tobacco Consumption: a discussion document reviewing the evidence.* Clive Smee, Chief Economic Adviser, Department of Health. DoH, London.
8 Department of Health (1991) *Children and Young Persons (Protection from Tobacco) Act.* HMSO, London.
9 Department of Health (1974) *Health and Safety at Work Act.* HMSO, London.
10 Carmelli D, Swan GE, Robinette D and Fabsitz R (1992) Genetic influence on smoking: a study of male twins. *NEJM.* **327**: 829–33.
11 Heath AC and Martin NG (1993) Genetic models for the natural history of smoking: evidence for a genetic influence on smoking persistence. *Addict Behav.* **18**: 19–34.

CHAPTER 2

Smoking and health

The fact that smoking is unhealthy is now well established in both the scientific and popular literature. Since the seminal work by Doll and Peto[1] and others in the USA in the 1950s that demonstrated the association between cigarette smoking and lung cancer, a number of epidemiological studies have provided evidence for an association between smoking and a variety of adverse effects of health. The increased mortality and morbidity in smokers is a consequence of the various components of cigarette smoke, and there is now a far clearer understanding of the biological basis of these associations.

One point is central – it is never too late to stop, regardless of the lifetime exposure to smoking or how late one stops.

Statistics and supporting evidence

Death attributable to smoking vs. number of deaths due to other causes[2]

Tobacco use has been implicated in the deaths of around 120 000 people in the UK every year, or about 330 deaths every day. This amounts to approximately 20% of all deaths. Around half of all regular cigarette smokers will die prematurely as a consequence of their smoking habit, and a quarter of regular smokers will die before the age of 70 years, losing on average 23 years of life. Smoking is the single largest cause of preventable illness and early death in the UK, dwarfing other causes such as road traffic accidents.

Certain diseases show a strong association with cigarette smoking, the latter being implicated in 80% of deaths from lung cancer, 80% of deaths from bronchitis and emphysema, and around 17% of deaths from coronary heart disease.

Table 2.1 Mortality and smoking in the UK

Condition	Deaths from condition attributable to smoking in 1995 (%)		Deaths from condition attributable to smoking in 1995 (number)		
	Men	Women	Men	Women	Total
Cancer					
Lung	90	73	21 100	9500	30 600
Throat/mouth	74	47	1500	400	1900
Oesophagus	71	62	2900	1600	4500
Bladder	48	17	1700	300	2000
Kidney	41	5	700	100	800
Stomach	35	10	1700	300	2000
Pancreas	21	25	600	800	1500
Unspecified	34	7	2400	500	3000
Leukaemia	19	10	200	100	300
Total					46 000
Cardiovascular diseases					
Ischaemic heart disease	23	11	18 700	7600	26 400
Aortic aneurysm	62	48	4000	1800	5800
Myocardial degeneration	24	10	300	300	600
Atherosclerosis	17	5	100	100	200
Stroke	13	9	3400	3900	7300
Total					40 300
Other					
Bronchitis/emphysema	86	79	15 100	9300	24 400
Pneumonia	25	11	5800	4100	9900
Stomach/duodenal ulcer	47	41	1000	1000	2000
Total					36 300
Total			81 300	41 700	123 000

Source: Action on Smoking and Health.[2]

Although there is evidence that smoking protects against the onset of a few diseases, specifically Parkinson's disease and endometrial cancer, the number of life-years gained is tiny by comparison with the number of life-years lost as a result of smoking in the population. The number of annual deaths that can be attributed to smoking is ten times greater than the number resulting from road traffic accidents and other accidental deaths.

Numbers admitted to NHS hospitals for treatment for smoking-related disease

The burden on the NHS caused by smoking-related disease is more difficult to quantify, since the figures quoted above relate only to smoking-related mortality and not to smoking-related morbidity. However, it is estimated that 284 000 patients are admitted to NHS hospitals every year with smoking-related disease, requiring 9500 hospital-bed spaces every day. The burden on primary care is equally large, with smoking-related disease and illness accounting for 8 million GP consultations and 7 million prescriptions annually.[3]

Box 2.1 Diseases and disorders for which smokers are at increased risk

Acute necrotising ulcerative
  gingivitis
Angina
Back pain
Buerger's disease
Carics
Cataract
Cataract, posterior subcapsular
Colon polyps
Crohn's disease
Depression
Diabetes (type 2)
Duodenal ulcer
Erectile dysfunction
Hearing loss
Impotence
Influenza

Ligament damage
Macular degeneration
Muscle damage
Nystagmus
Ocular histoplasmosis
Optic neuropathy
Osteoarthritis
Osteoporosis
Peripheral vascular disease
Pneumonia
Psoriasis
Rheumatoid arthritis
Skin wrinkling
Stomach ulcer
Tendon damage
Tobacco amblyopia
Tuberculosis

Source: Action on Smoking and Health.[2]

Box 2.2 Increased severity of disease or symptoms in smokers

Asthma	Graves' disease
Chronic rhinitis	Influenza
Common cold	Multiple sclerosis
Crohn's disease	Optic neurosis
Diabetic retinopathy	Pneumonia
	Tuberculosis

Source: Action on Smoking and Health.[2]

Box 2.3 Functional impairment in smokers

Ejaculation	Sperm count
Fertility	Sperm motility
Immune function	Sperm penetration of ovum
Menopause	Sperm shape

Source: Action on Smoking and Health.[2]

Common diseases caused by smoking

The earliest observations that smoking has a detrimental impact on health can be traced back almost as far as the introduction of the habit to Western society in the fifteenth and sixteenth centuries (*see* Chapter 1). However, more rigorous evidence for the association between smoking (particularly, but not exclusively, of cigarettes) and specific diseases has become available during the last 50 years. Nicotine itself is highly poisonous (it is used as an insecticide, and 60 mg would be sufficient to kill if taken orally in pure form). However, it is the other constituents of cigarette smoke, in particular the constituents of tar, that cause the greatest damage. The length of time for which an individual has smoked, rather than the amount, is most important in determining the level of risk, so delaying initiation could also be important.

Cancers

Approximately 30% of deaths from cancers of all kinds can be attributed to cigarette smoking. In particular, there is now convincing

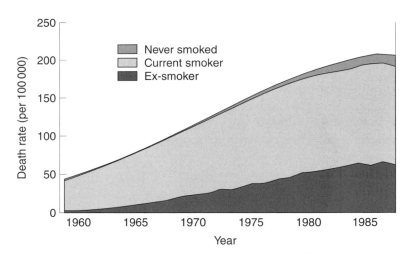

Figure 2.1: Contribution to white male lung cancer rates by smoking status, for the birth cohort 1910–14.
Source: Smoking and Tobacco Control Monograph No. 13, National Cancer Institute, Bethesda, MD.

evidence that smoking is associated with the development of several specific cancers, and the nature of this association is becoming increasingly understood at the cellular level. This has been shown to be primarily a consequence of the components of the particulate phase of tobacco smoke. It is less clear whether, after the development of some (smoking-related and other) cancers, persistent smoking makes a difference to *survival*. It seems likely that it does so, at the very least, although it is not yet known whether there are effects on cancer progression and recurrence that affect survival, and how this may vary according to site.

Lung

Almost a quarter of cancer deaths are due to lung cancer, which makes it the commonest form of cancer death, and the vast majority of these cases are associated with smoking. Mortality from lung cancer decreased by almost a third between the mid-1980s and the mid-1990s, continuing a trend that had begun in the 1970s and which has mirrored the decline in smoking prevalence in the population. Almost a quarter of those who die as a result of smoking will die from lung cancer, although the risk of lung cancer associated with smoking begins to decrease as soon as the smoker stops, eventually declining to almost the risk for someone who has never smoked. There is a weak dose–response relationship between the number of cigarettes smoked per day and mortality from lung cancer. Light smokers who smoke between one and 14 cigarettes a day have an eightfold higher risk of death from lung cancer compared with non-smokers, while heavy smokers who smoke 25 or more cigarettes a day have a 25-fold higher risk compared with non-smokers. Individual differences in the metabolism of nicotine, and consequently in the amount of smoke (and therefore tar) that is inhaled in order to achieve a certain blood level of nicotine, account for the relative weakness of this dose–response relationship.

Cervix

There is now considerable evidence for an association between cigarette smoking and cervical cancer, although it remains unclear whether this is a causal association or whether it is due to indirect confounding factors, such as the association of smoking with the number of sexual partners. However, there is evidence for changes in the cervical mucus of smokers compared with non-smokers (e.g. the presence of biogenic amines such as cotinine), which supports a causal association.

Pancreas

Pancreatic cancer is an aggressive cancer with very low survival rates, and it has been shown to be associated with smoking status, being related to both cigarette consumption and duration of smoking. The relative risk in smokers falls to that in non-smokers approximately ten years after cessation.

Kidney and bladder

There is evidence for an association between smoking and both kidney and bladder cancer, with smokers having approximately twice the risk of developing kidney cancer compared with non-smokers. Early initiation of smoking also appears to contribute to the risk of kidney cancer.

Oral (including mouth, lip, tongue and throat)

Cigarette smoking, as well as pipe and cigar smoking, is a risk factor for all oral cancers (i.e. those associated with the larynx, oral cavity and oesophagus). The vast majority of patients with oral cancer are tobacco users, although the delivery device may include cigarettes, pipe, cigars, chewing tobacco and others. This risk increases as tobacco consumption increases, and there is also evidence for an interactive contribution of alcohol to the risk of oral cancer among smokers. Smoking is the major contributing factor in the majority of cancers of the oral cavity, larynx and oesophagus.

Leukaemia

There is strong evidence for an association between cigarette smoking and leukaemia, and this relationship becomes stronger as the number of cigarettes smoked increases. The risk is reduced in ex-smokers (1.39 compared with 1.53 for current smokers).

Breast

Breast cancer has been shown to be associated with both active smoking and long-term passive smoking, although there is only limited published evidence available at present.

Anus

Recent evidence suggests that there is an association between cigarette smoking and anal cancer in premenopausal women, with a dose-dependent relationship being reported between the number of pack-years (where 1 pack-year is defined as 20 cigarettes/day per year) and risk of anal cancer.

Coronary heart disease, thrombosis, atherosclerosis, stroke and Buerger's disease

Coronary heart disease is a general term that refers to the interruption or diminution of the normal supply of blood to the heart through the coronary arteries. This may occur either as a result of the gradual build-up of fatty deposits, resulting in eventual blockage (atherosclerosis), or as a consequence of the formation of a blood clot in an artery (thrombosis – it is rarely embolic). Cigarette smoking is the most important modifiable, non-genetic risk factor for coronary heart disease, with the risk for a smoker being two to three times greater than the corresponding risk for a non-smoker. This has been shown to be primarily due to the components of the vapour phase of tobacco smoke, including carbon monoxide. Approximately 17% of all deaths from heart disease can be accounted for by smoking, this figure being unevenly split between men (23% of all heart disease deaths) and women (11% of all heart disease deaths). This includes myocardial infarction (heart attack) and cerebral thrombosis (stroke). Approximately 11% of all deaths from stroke are associated with smoking. Smoking low-tar cigarettes does not seem to reduce the risk significantly. Among individuals with existing coronary disease, the severity of the disease is far greater in smokers than in non-smokers.

The inhalation of tobacco smoke causes an immediate increase in heart rate (about 5–10 beats/minute even in tolerant smokers) and blood pressure (2–5 mmHg systolic), with the carbon monoxide component having an immediate impact on the oxygen-carrying capacity of the blood. However, more important in the aetiology of coronary heart disease is the fact that smoking results in an increase in blood cholesterol levels, raised levels of fibrinogen and increased platelet counts. As the atherosclerotic disease process progresses the arteries become increasingly narrow and rigid, while the blood becomes increasingly likely to form a thrombosis (i.e. a clot) as a result of increased platelet counts and fibrinogen levels. This increases the likelihood of a subsequent heart attack or stroke. Following clinical disease (e.g. myocardial infarction), the risk of further events and death *declines* once smoking has ceased.

Other vascular risks that are increased in smokers include aneurysm, in which the arterial wall weakens and expands, leading to an increased risk of bursting or clotting. Smokers also have a dramatically increased risk of developing peripheral vascular disease in the limbs and extremities, which in severe cases can result in gangrene and amputation. A rare form of this is Buerger's disease (thromboangiitis obliterans), which affects the small and medium-sized arteries, veins and nerves of the arms and legs. Symptoms are usually detectable at a relatively early age (before 45 years).

Chronic bronchitis, emphysema and other lung/airway disease

Approximately 20% of all smoking-related deaths each year are due to chronic obstructive lung disease, such as chronic bronchitis and emphysema. These are progressively disabling diseases that can cause prolonged suffering as a result of the gradual obstruction and narrowing of the small airways in the lungs and the simultaneous destruction of air sacs in the lungs. Although most individuals with lung cancer do not survive for more than one year after diagnosis, the quality of life of individuals with chronic obstructive lung disease can deteriorate over a substantial time period. The increasing breathlessness often only becomes recognised as a problem by the affected individual after approximately half of the lung has been destroyed.

Over 80% of deaths due to chronic obstructive lung disease can be attributed to smoking, so the condition is rare in non-smokers. There is a direct relationship between the number of cigarettes smoked and the risk of death from this disease.

Pneumonia is more common among smokers, and it is also more likely to prove fatal than in non-smokers. Figures from 1995 suggest that almost 10 000 deaths that year from pneumonia could be attributed to smoking.[2]

Other disorders

Women who smoke while taking the contraceptive pill have a tenfold higher risk of coronary heart disease than women who take the contraceptive pill but do not smoke. Cigarette smoking has also been associated with increased risk of infertility in women, and with subfertility in both men and women. Women who are regular smokers are also more likely to have an earlier menopause than non-smoking women. On average, women who are smokers become menopausal two years earlier than women who are non-smokers, and they are more likely to suffer from osteoporosis subsequently.

Smoking is also associated with a number of other effects that may be regarded as health problems, including the following:

- impaired sense of taste and smell
- increased facial wrinkles, at an earlier age
- poor dental hygiene
- stomach ulcers
- longer wound-healing times.

There is also a strong association between cigarette smoking and a number of psychiatric disorders, such as anxiety disorders, depression and schizophrenia. However, the direction of causation in these cases is an important issue. For example, the vast majority of schizophrenic individuals are smokers, but it is not suggested that cigarette smoking *causes* schizophrenia. Rather, in this case, it has been suggested that smoking in schizophrenics represents a form of self-medication to allow them to manage their symptoms. Antipsychotic medication may also result in increased smoking in order to manage the side-effects of the medication. In the case of depression, the situation is similarly complex, and it has been suggested that this association arises from a genetic risk that predisposes to both smoking behaviour and depression, or that smoking is also self-medication in this case.

It is true that mean stress levels are higher in smokers than in non-smokers, and smokers may continue their habit at least partly as a means of coping with stress. However, there is evidence that higher levels of stress decrease once an individual has stopped smoking, which suggests that the subjective stress experienced by smokers and apparently combated by smoking may in fact be a consequence of smoking itself.

Finally, smoking has been shown to have a protective effect against Parkinson's disease, possibly through the effect of nicotine on dopamine neurotransmission. There is also some weaker evidence that smoking has a protective effect against Alzheimer's disease, although any benefits associated with smoking are far outweighed by the attendant risks.

Pregnancy and childbirth

Smoking during pregnancy has been associated with an increased risk of spontaneous abortion, haemorrhage, premature birth and low birth weight, as well as a number of problems following the birth of the infant, such as respiratory illness, chronic cough and wheezing, chronic middle ear effusion (glue ear) and sudden infant death syndrome. Whether smoking reduces the risk of pre-eclampsia is uncertain.

Many pregnant women continue to smoke during the course of their pregnancy, while others are aware of the risks associated with smoking during pregnancy, and do attempt to stop. However, of those that succeed, a large proportion return to their smoking habit following childbirth, thereby exposing the infant to the risks of passive smoking. In addition, the partners of pregnant smokers usually continue to smoke. This has the effect of reducing the likelihood of the mother's attempt to stop being successful, as well as contributing to the ambient smoke to which the pregnant woman and subsequently the infant are exposed. There is some weak evidence that exposure of the mother to passive smoking during pregnancy is associated with a higher risk of spontaneous abortion and a lower than average birth weight.

Fertility

There is now substantial evidence that smoking has a detrimental effect on fertility, with an association between smoking and both

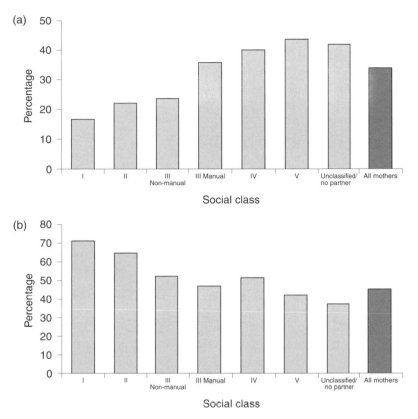

Figure 2.2: (a) Percentage of women in England who smoked before or during pregnancy. (b) Percentage of women in England who gave up smoking before or during pregnancy.
Source: Infant Feeding Survey 2000; BMRB Social Research.[4]

infertility and subfertility. There is also evidence for an association between smoking and infertility, subfertility and impotence in men who smoke. For example, the increased risk of impotence is 50% in men aged between 30 and 40 years.

Furthermore, the rate of spontaneous abortion is higher in women who are smokers than in those who are non-smokers. Other risks that are increased in pregnant women who are smokers include haemorrhaging during pregnancy, premature detachment of the placenta and premature rupture of the membranes.

Premature birth and low birth weight

The risk of premature birth is also increased among women who smoke, and babies born to smokers are on average 200 g lighter than those born to non-smokers (when other factors are controlled for). This is in turn associated with an increased risk of morbidity and mortality during early infancy. This risk is primarily associated with smoking in the second and third trimesters of pregnancy. Thus stopping smoking during the first trimester reduces the risk to the fetus almost to the level for the fetus of a non-smoking mother.

Acute respiratory illness

Infants born to families in which one or both parents smoke are more likely to suffer from acute respiratory illness than those who are born to non-smoking families. This will be discussed in more detail in the section on the effects of passive smoking.

Passive smoking

In recent years there has been growing concern about the risks to non-smokers associated with exposure to the 'second-hand' smoke generated by smokers. Until recently there was limited evidence to quantify the degree of risk, if any, associated with passive smoking, not least because it is difficult to quantify the degree of exposure. However, a picture is now emerging of health risks associated with passive smoking, albeit on a much reduced scale compared with the risks of active smoking. This concern, and the growing body of evidence to support some association between passive smoking and illness, combined with the growing social unacceptability of smoking to many people, has resulted in an increasing number of smoke-free public places, such as hospitals, schools, places of entertainment, and so on.

Definition

Passive smoking can be defined as exposure to environmental tobacco smoke – that is, the mixture of effluents that is directly released into the ambient air between puffs during smoking of the tobacco product, or exhaled by the smoker. Cigarette smoke consists of 'mainstream' smoke, which is drawn along the cigarette tube through the filter and inhaled, and 'sidestream' smoke, which is burned off the tip of the cigarette. Sidestream smoke contains a higher proportion of tar and other harmful products than mainstream smoke, as the latter passes through the filter. The majority of ambient smoke around a smoker is sidestream smoke, and it is primarily this to which non-smokers are exposed during passive smoking.

Links with health problems

There is growing evidence that passive smoking adversely affects the health of infants and young children in particular, increasing the risk of lower respiratory tract infection, chronic cough, wheezing, sudden infant death syndrome and chronic middle ear effusion (glue ear), as well as exacerbating the severity of asthma symptoms. For example, there is evidence that children reared in families where both parents smoke have a 72% increased risk for respiratory illness compared with children raised in non-smoking families.

More recent research also indicates that passive smoking is associated with an increased risk of heart disease in adults, with non-smokers exposed to passive smoking showing a 23% increase in the risk of coronary heart disease compared with non-smokers not exposed in this way. However, other studies have failed to show a clear association, and it is possible that misclassification of smoking status (i.e. smokers not admitting to their smoking habit) may be an important source of bias in such studies.

There is also evidence that passive smoking is associated with an increased risk of lung cancer. For example, the overall increase in risk found across six European studies was 45% for non-smokers living with smokers, compared with couples where both individuals were non-smokers. In a series of studies in the USA, women who had never smoked but who lived with smokers had a 20% higher risk of developing lung cancer than similar women who lived with non-smokers. The absolute level of risk remains low, but this increase in risk among individuals who are exposed to passive smoke provides evidence for the adverse effects of passive smoking. However, once again other studies have failed to show any association, and it is important to be aware of the methodological difficulties inherent in any attempt to calculate the level of risk associated with passive smoking.

In adults there is some evidence for an association between passive smoking and increased eye, nose and throat irritation, reduced lung function and exacerbation of asthma symptoms.

It has been estimated that 17 000 admissions of young children (under the age of 5 years) to hospital every year are a consequence of exposure to passive smoking, often in the home environment as a result of one or both parents smoking.[2] However, any assessment of the impact of passive smoking requires accurate estimates of the increase in risk of specific diseases associated with passive smoking. This is premature, given the ongoing debate on this topic. However, it is probably safe to say that young children are at higher risk than adults, and that the increased risk in adults will be at worst modest compared with the risks of active smoking.

It is difficult to estimate the later impact of respiratory disease in infancy, but it is possible that it may contribute to subsequent respiratory disease in adulthood.

Smoking cessation

The reasons for stopping smoking are well documented, and the preceding summary highlights the various risks – some well known

Table 2.2 Health benefits of stopping smoking

Time since stopping	Beneficial health changes
20 minutes	Blood pressure and pulse rate return to normal
8 hours	Blood nicotine and carbon monoxide levels decrease by 50%, and oxygen levels return to normal
24 hours	Carbon monoxide will be eliminated from the body; lungs start to clear out mucus and other smoking debris
48 hours	There is no nicotine left in the body; ability to taste and smell is greatly improved
72 hours	Breathing becomes easier; bronchial tubes begin to relax and energy levels increase
2–12 weeks	Circulation improves
3–9 months	Coughing, wheezing and breathing problems improve as lung function is increased by up to 10%
1 year	Risk of a heart attack falls to about 50% of that of a smoker
10 years	Risk of lung cancer falls to 50% of that of a smoker
15 years	Risk of a heart attack falls to the same level as in someone who has never smoked

and others less so – of continued smoking. The counterpoint to this, and one that it is important to emphasise to those who are considering attempting to stop, is that the health *benefits* of stopping begin immediately (*see* Table 2.2).

Smoking cessation will be associated with varying degrees of withdrawal (*see* Table 2.3).

Although many smokers report an increase in anxiety when they stop smoking, current evidence suggests that rather than being a withdrawal symptom, this anxiety is generated by the actual act of trying to stop smoking. Those individuals who successfully abstain for four weeks report a significant reduction in anxiety to below baseline levels.

Of course, although the broad symptoms and signs associated with withdrawal are similar in most smokers who stop, the degree of severity varies substantially. This presents an interesting challenge to understanding nicotine addiction, and may also offer some scope

Table 2.3 Withdrawal symptoms and signs associated with smoking cessation

Symptom	Duration	Prevalence
Irritability/aggression	< 4 weeks	50%
Depression	< 4 weeks	60%
Restlessness	< 4 weeks	60%
Impaired concentration	< 2 weeks	60%
Increased appetite	< 10 weeks	70%
Light-headedness	< 48 hours	10%
Sleep disturbance	< 1 week	25%
Craving	> 2 weeks	70%
Sign	*Duration*	*Prevalence*
Decrease in heart rate	Long term	> 80%
Decreased adrenaline release	Short term	Not known
Decreased cortisol release	< 4 weeks	Not known
Increased alpha-wave EEG output	Not known	Not known
Reduced dominant alpha frequency in EEG output	Not known	Not known
Decreased tremor	Long term	> 80%
Decreased resting metabolic rate	Long term	Not known
Increased skin temperature	Long term	> 80%
Decreased salivary immunoglobulin A	< 14 days	Not known
Decreased caffeine metabolism	Long term	> 80%
Increased weight	Long term	> 80%

Source: West.[5]

for the future tailoring of pharmacological interventions to individuals. In addition, some of these signs and symptoms present far more of a challenge than others to those who are attempting to quit. For example, weight gain is a particular problem associated with relapse (especially in women). Cravings are unusual in that they can persist for far longer than the typical four weeks of withdrawal symptoms usually cited, and they are frequently triggered by environmental cues, such as the sight of a packet of cigarettes, or a location (e.g. a pub) that is strongly associated with smoking. Learning to identify and thus avoid such cues can be a useful behavioural adjunct to cessation attempts.

Reflection exercises

Exercise 2

Do you know the mortality and morbidity rates associated with smoking? Do you know how individuals from different socio-economic groups fare? If you do not know these statistics for your patient population, then find out more from your local public health department or statistical reference tables.

Exercise 3

Ask ten consecutive patients who are cigarette smokers who consult you to describe what risks they perceive they have of developing smoking-related conditions such as coronary heart disease or stroke, or other consequences of smoking, such as cancers. Do they have realistic perspectives? What educational tools would be useful to inform them about the risks? Ask your local health education unit for help.

Exercise 4

Undertake an audit to determine the proportion of individuals with diabetes in your patient population who have a history of smoking recorded. Randomly select 20 case notes of people with type 1 and type 2 diabetes for this exercise.

(i) What proportion have had their smoking status recorded during the last year?

(ii) How can this proportion be improved? Draw up an action plan and re-audit in 12 months' time.

(iii) Do you know which interventions for smoking cessation are most likely to be successful, and for which patients with diabetes they are warranted? How could you target these patients? Draw up an action plan for the interventions to be introduced in the monitoring system for patients with diabetes.

Now that you have completed this interactive reflection exercise, transfer the information to the empty template of the personal development plan on pages 169–178 if you are working on your own learning plan, or to the practice personal and professional development plan on pages 193–199 if you are working on a practice team learning plan. Don't forget to keep the evidence of your learning in your personal portfolio.

References

1 Doll R and Richard P (1976) Mortality in relation to smoking: 20 years' observation on male British doctors. *BMJ.* **2**: 1525–36.

2 Action on Smoking and Health (2002) http://www.ash.org.uk/.

3 Godfrey and Maynard (1988) Economic aspects of tobacco use and taxation policy. *BMJ.* **297**: 339–43.

4 *Infant Feeding 2000* – a survey conducted on behalf of the Department of Health, the Scottish Executive, the National Assembly for Wales and the Department of Health, Social Services and Public Safety in Northern Ireland.

5 West R (1999) Psychological effects of nicotine and smoking in man. In: *Nicotine Addiction in Britain.* Royal College of Physicians, London.

CHAPTER 3

Psychological and behavioural techniques

Psychological and behavioural techniques

As with any addiction, the motivational and behavioural aspects play a key role in the success of any cessation attempt and in the prevention of relapse. For example, self-efficacy beliefs (defined as the extent to which the individual feels capable of successfully stopping smoking) are a strong predictor of initial success and the subsequent avoidance of relapse.

In addition, the psychological aspects of withdrawal, such as cravings, biases in attention towards smoking-related cues, and the intrusion of thoughts and images related to smoking, can be minimised by the use of thought-suppression techniques such as distraction. Many well-established smoking cessation programmes include elements that implicitly rely on these techniques, which have been developed from general principles and applied for many years.

A number of techniques may be of value. Some can be recommended on the basis of comparison with placebo, while some may simply help (if the smoker wishes to try them) as an extension of the influence of the therapist advising and assisting cessation, and reinforcing existing motivation rather than as an additional aid. Against this may be set any demoralising consequences that arise from trying and failing. The systematic reviews of the Cochrane Tobacco Addiction Review Group are relied upon by the Society for Research on Nicotine and Tobacco (SRNT) and the World Health Organisation (WHO) when making authoritative statements about the efficacy of various interventions.

Individual interventions

Individual behavioural counselling

Individual behavioural counselling requires a number of processes and skills, most of which are possessed by healthcare professionals as a result of their daily activities, such as appropriate greetings, eliciting relevant information, directing the conversation, and so on. Other important aspects include the following:

- establishing a rapport with the patients
- clear, unambiguous conversation
- calibrating the conversation and checking the patient's understanding
- providing directions and correcting errors
- summarising information to be remembered
- maintaining a positive tone.

This is much more directive and goal oriented than more typical counselling approaches. The following points should be raised, preferably during the course of several consultations that take place over the duration of the cessation attempt.

- Explain how nicotine replacement therapy (NRT) and Zyban can help, and the limitations of these aids.
- Explain the withdrawal symptoms (what to expect, how long they will last, etc.).
- Explain that a quit date should be set, and that smoking should continue as normal until this date.
- Offer the patient help in preparing for this date (reasons for stopping, completing a 'declaration' card, etc.).
- Give practical advice on preparation for this date (getting rid of all cigarettes, cues to smoking, etc.).
- Maintain contact with the patient (possibly by telephone) before, on and following the quit date.

During this period of contact, the focus should be on maintaining motivation, discussing difficulties that have been encountered, providing advice on coping with these problems, and congratulating success. For example:

- discussing withdrawal discomfort and explaining why this occurs
- emphasising the importance of total abstinence
- explaining the difference between a *lapse* and a *relapse.*

If the attempt fails, the patient should be advised to wait for a few months before the next attempt, and to use the present, failed attempt to identify obstacles and develop strategies for overcoming them.

If behavioural support is to be offered, the following points must be addressed initially:

- identification of smoking behaviour
- assessment of the level of readiness to attempt cessation
- provision of information.

Butler *et al.*[1] have described the following method of motivational consulting, in which the aim is to build the patient's motivation and confidence with regard to stopping smoking.

1 The patient is invited to rate numerically their motivation and confidence with regard to stopping smoking.
2 The clinician responds to these scores using specific questions and strategies.
3 The patient is invited to set meaningful targets for him- or herself.

The counselling interventions typically included the following components: review of a participant's smoking history and motivation to quit, help in the identification of high-risk situations, and the generation of problem-solving strategies to deal with such situaions. Counsellors may also have provided non-specific support and encouragement. Additional components such as written materials, video or audiotapes may also have been provided.

There is consistent evidence that individual counselling increases the likelihood of cessation compared to less intensive support. Whilst most of the trials were undertaken in hospitalised smokers, counselling was also shown to be effective in a workplace setting[2] and amongst community volunteers.

Lancaster and Stead[3]

Thus brief advice and support have been shown to be effective, but more intensive support and follow-up improve success rates even further.

Aversive smoking

Aversive smoking refers to the practice of pairing the act of smoking with an aversive stimulus so that, by a process of associated learning,

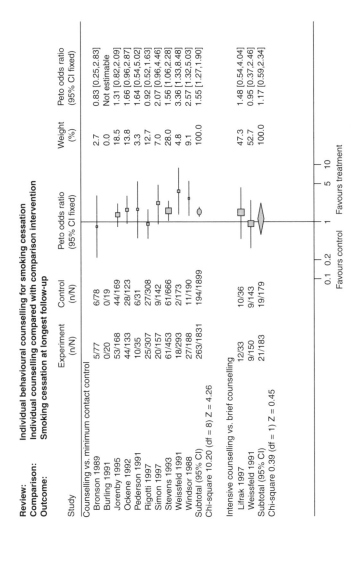

Review:	Individual behavioural counselling for smoking cessation
Comparison:	Individual counselling compared with comparison intervention
Outcome:	Smoking cessation at longest follow-up

Study	Experiment (n/N)	Control (n/N)	Peto odds ratio (95% CI fixed)	Weight (%)	Peto odds ratio (95% CI fixed)
Counselling vs. minimum contact control					
Bronson 1989	5/77	6/78		2.7	0.83 [0.25,2.83]
Burling 1991	0/20	0/19		0.0	Not estimable
Jorenby 1995	53/168	44/169		18.5	1.31 [0.82,2.09]
Ockene 1992	44/133	28/123		13.8	1.66 [0.96,2.87]
Pederson 1991	10/35	6/31		3.3	1.64 [0.54,5.02]
Rigotti 1997	25/307	27/308		12.7	0.92 [0.52,1.63]
Simon 1997	20/157	9/142		7.0	2.07 [0.96,4.46]
Stevens 1993	61/453	61/666		28.0	1.56 [1.06,2.28]
Weissfeld 1991	18/293	2/173		4.8	3.36 [1.33,8.48]
Windsor 1988	27/188	11/190		9.1	2.57 [1.32,5.03]
Subtotal (95% CI)	263/1831	194/1899		100.0	1.55 [1.27,1.90]
Chi-square 10.20 (df = 8) Z = 4.26					
Intensive counselling vs. brief counselling					
Lifrak 1997	12/33	10/36		47.3	1.48 [0.54,4.04]
Weissfeld 1991	9/150	9/143		52.7	0.95 [0.37,2.46]
Subtotal (95% CI)	21/183	19/179		100.0	1.17 [0.59,2.34]
Chi-square 0.39 (df = 1) Z = 0.45					

0.1 0.2   1   5 10

Favours control   Favours treatment

Figure 3.1: Findings with regard to individual behavioural counselling for smoking cessation.[3]

the act of smoking itself becomes aversive. For example, this intervention may involve requiring the smoker to smoke very rapidly (over-smoke) so that an overdose of nicotine results, with accompanying aversive symptoms.

> The existing studies provide insufficient evidence of the efficacy of rapid smoking. A dose-response to aversion stimulation has not been clearly demonstrated, but existing data do not allow an unequivocal conclusion here either. Milder versions of 'aversion smoking' seem ineffective.
>
> In the current era of pharmacological treatments for smoking, research in behavioural methods has declined considerably, despite the acknowledged need for behavioural accompaniments to drug therapies. Rapid smoking remains an unproven method with sufficient indications of promise to warrant evaluation using modern rigorous methodology.
>
> Hajek and Stead[4]

Exercise

Exercise has been shown to provide treatment benefits for a range of conditions, such as mild clinical depression.

> Only one of the eight trials reviewed offered evidence for exercise aiding smoking cessation. However, the trials which did not show a significant effect of exercise on smoking abstinence were too small to exclude reliably an effect of intervention and had numerous methodological limitations. There is insufficient evidence to recommend exercise as a specific aid to smoking cessation.
>
> Ussher et al.[5]

However, although exercise itself may not be an effective smoking cessation aid, sports organisations may be used to promote smoking cessation as part of an integrated tobacco control programme. In certain community-based initiatives this has included visits by well-known sportsmen (footballers, etc.) to schools to promote (among other things) non-smoking. Increased exercise levels may also help to offset any increase in weight which typically accompanies smoking cessation.

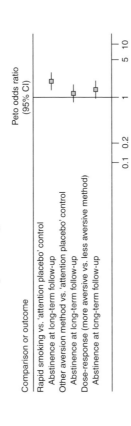

Figure 3.2: Findings with regard to aversive smoking for smoking cessation. [4]

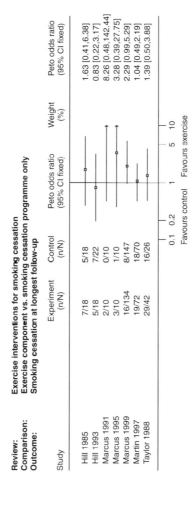

Figure 3.3: Findings with regard to exercise interventions for smoking cessation.[5]

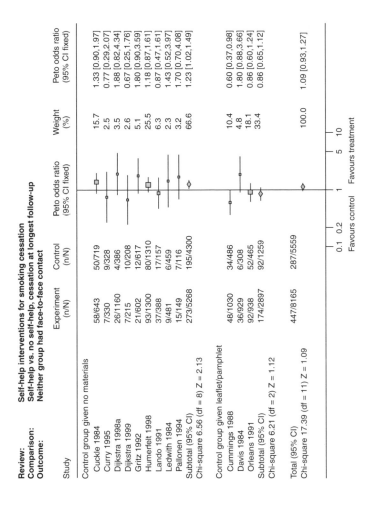

Review:	Self-help interventions for smoking cessation
Comparison:	Self-help vs. no self-help, cessation at longest follow-up
Outcome:	Neither group had face-to-face contact

Study	Experiment (n/N)	Control (n/N)	Peto odds ratio (95% CI fixed)	Weight (%)	Peto odds ratio (95% CI fixed)
Control group given no materials					
Cuckle 1984	58/643	50/719		15.7	1.33 [0.90,1.97]
Curry 1995	7/330	9/328		2.5	0.77 [0.29,2.07]
Dijkstra 1998a	26/1160	4/386		3.5	1.88 [0.82,4.34]
Dijkstra 1999	7/215	10/208		2.6	0.67 [0.25,1.76]
Gritz 1992	21/602	12/617		5.1	1.80 [0.90,3.59]
Humerfelt 1998	93/1300	80/1310		25.5	1.18 [0.87,1.61]
Lando 1991	37/388	17/157		6.3	0.87 [0.47,1.61]
Ledwith 1984	9/481	6/459		2.3	1.43 [0.52,3.97]
Pallonen 1994	15/149	7/116		3.2	1.70 [0.70,4.08]
Subtotal (95% CI)	273/5268	195/4300		66.6	1.23 [1.02,1.49]
Chi-square 6.56 (df = 8) Z = 2.13					
Control group given leaflet/pamphlet					
Cummings 1988	48/1030	34/486		10.4	0.60 [0.37,0.98]
Davis 1984	36/929	6/308		4.8	1.80 [0.88,3.66]
Orleans 1991	92/938	52/465		18.1	0.86 [0.60,1.24]
Subtotal (95% CI)	174/2897	92/1259		33.4	0.86 [0.65,1.12]
Chi-square 6.21 (df = 2) Z = 1.12					
Total (95% CI)	447/8165	287/5559		100.0	1.09 [0.93,1.27]
Chi-square 17.39 (df = 11) Z = 1.09					

0.1 0.2   1   5 10
Favours control   Favours treatment

Figure 3.4: Findings with regard to self-help interventions for smoking cessation.[6]

Self-help interventions

A major limitation of therapist-delivered behavioural interventions is that they reach only a small proportion of smokers. Most successful quitters give up on their own. Methods for supporting otherwise unaided quit attempts therefore have the potential to help a far greater proportion of the smoking population.

> Access to information, in understandable formats, is important for individuals who smoke, as it is for those with other kinds of medical problem. This review examined the specific effect of materials which aimed to provide a structured approach to smoking cessation beyond simple information. Such materials may provide a very small increase in quitting compared to no intervention. There is no evidence that self-help materials produce incremental benefits over other minimal interventions, such as advice from a healthcare professional, or nicotine replacement therapy. There is increasing evidence that materials tailored for individual smokers are more effective.
>
> Lancaster and Stead[6]

Self-help materials are usually in the form of written materials (including quitting diaries, etc.), but may take the form of other media, such as audio- and videotapes. Tailoring can take the form of a personalised plan, which is offered with some NRT products, such as NiQuitin CQ.

Telephone counselling

QUIT is a UK non-governmental organisation dedicated to helping smokers stop. It provides the Quitline telephone helpline service, which is staffed by qualified counsellors trained in smoking cessation. It was launched in 1990 and has recently expanded to include Quitlines in various languages (Bengali, Gujurati, Hindi, Punjabi, Urdu, etc.) and a Pregnancy Quitline. Since 1995 it has been funded by the Health Education Authority, which allows Quitline to operate as a freephone service, so that by 1997 Quitline was receiving 500000 calls annually. The service also offers a 'call-back' facility to any UK landline, to encourage those on limited incomes to use the service.

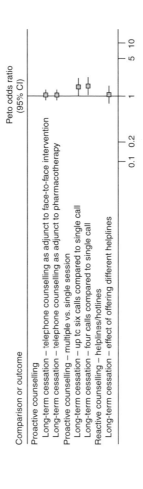

Figure 3.5: Findings with regard to telephone counselling for smoking cessation.[7]

As the main component of an intervention, proactive telephone counselling helps smokers to quit. Although the size of effect is uncertain, a call from a counsellor is likely to increase the chances of quitting. Reactive counselling via telephone helplines has not been evaluated in the same way, but indirect evidence suggests that callers receiving counselling via a quitline also have an increased chance of successfully quitting. Telephone quitlines provide an important route of access to support for smokers, and call-back counselling may enhance their usefulness. Telephone counselling as follow-up to a face-to-face intervention may lead to a small increase in success rates compared to face-to-face intervention alone, but the evidence for this effect is weaker.

Stead and Lancaster[7]

Group interventions

Although the majority of smokers attempt to give up either completely unaided or with individual support, pharmacological therapy, etc., there is growing evidence that group interventions are of *additional* benefit.

Community intervention

Community-based initiatives focus on specific groups within a community (e.g. women, ethnic communities, etc.), and attempt to raise awareness of smoking-related issues and promote cessation by increasing the accessibility of support mechanisms. This can be extended to include smoke-free initiatives in schools, businesses and other places, education in schools, and so on.

Community interventions are defined here as co-ordinated, widespread programmes which support non-smoking behaviour in a particular geographical area (e.g. school districts) or region, or in groupings of people who share common interests or needs.

Overall, there is some limited support for the effectiveness of community interventions in preventing the uptake of smoking in young people.[8] GP intervention also delays the uptake of smoking in young people.

The following programme characteristics could be considered by individuals involved in planning future community programmes.

- Elements of existing programmes that have been shown to be effective should be built on, rather than repeating methods that have achieved limited success.
- Programmes need to be flexible enough to accommodate the variability between communities, so that the different components of a given programme can be modified to achieve acceptability in different contexts.
- Developmental work should be carried out with representative samples of those individuals to be targeted, so that appropriate messages and activities can be implemented.
- Programme messages and activities should be guided by theoretical constructs about the way in which behaviours are acquired and maintained (e.g. social learning theory).
- Community activities must reach the intended audience if they are to have any chance of successfully influencing the behaviour of that audience.

Group behavioural counselling

A growing number of multi-component, intensive smoking cessation services are available, targeted in particular at smokers who have tried and failed to give up several times previously. The effectiveness of such group programmes must therefore be considered in the light of the fact that most participants are likely to be highly dependent smokers. There is some support for the notion that the group support component of such programmes constitutes an 'active ingredient' in its own right that improves the response of the smoker beyond that to simple advice.

> There is reasonable evidence that groups are better than self-help and other less intensive interventions, although they may be no better than advice from a healthcare provider. There is not enough evidence on their effectiveness compared to intensive individual counselling. From the point of view of the consumer who is motivated to make a quit attempt, it is probably worth joining a group if one is available – it will increase the likelihood of quitting. Group therapy may also be valuable as part of a comprehensive intervention which includes NRT.
>
> From the public health perspective, the impact of groups on smoking prevalence will depend on their uptake. Providers need to make a judgement about the cost-effectiveness of the gains achieved by group therapy compared to other interventions.
>
> Stead and Lancaster[9]

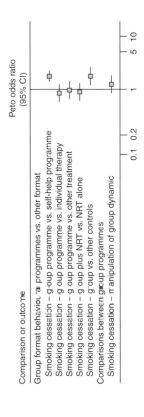

Figure 3.6: Findings with regard to group behaviour therapy programmes for smoking cessation.[9]

Individual differences in efficacy

Personality

Although there is substantial evidence that personality plays a role in mediating the initiation of smoking (but less evidence suggesting a role for it in the maintenance of smoking), there does not seem to be any association between personality and the success of smoking cessation attempts in general, or between personality and the efficacy of different smoking cessation interventions.

Psychiatric diagnosis

There is evidence for an association between depression and smoking – smoking is common among those with a current or past history of depression. In at least one study, smokers with a history of major depression were found to have an increased likelihood of experiencing another episode of major depression in the period following a successful smoking cessation attempt.

It is also known that the prevalence of smoking in individuals with a diagnosis of schizophrenia is extremely high (over 90%), and this is thought to be due to an attempt at self-medication, either to ameliorate the symptoms of the disease or to reduce the aversive side-effects of antipsychotic medication. This has typically resulted in low cessation rates among individuals in this group.

Timing of interventions to maximise effect

Teachable moments

A 'teachable moment' is simply any opportunity that arises to bring up a topic – in this case smoking cessation – when the recipient of the message is in a state that maximises the impact and accessibility of the message. Most obviously, contact with a health professional when health issues are the topic of discussion represents one such teachable

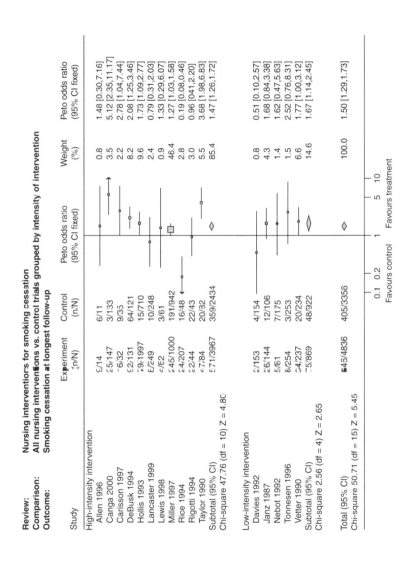

Figure 3.7: Findings with regard to nursing interventions for smoking cessation.[10]

moment, especially if the reason for the consultation is related to smoking.

Nursing interventions

> The results of this review indicate the potential benefits of intervention given by nurses to their patients. The challenge will be to incorporate smoking cessation intervention as part of standard practice so that all patients are given an opportunity to be queried about their tobacco use and to be given advice to quit along with reinforcement and follow-up. Nicotine replacement therapy [and Zyban] has been shown to improve quit rates when used in conjunction with counselling for behavioural change, and should be considered an important adjunct, but not a replacement, for nursing intervention.
>
> Rice and Stead[10]

It should be borne in mind that although a moment may be 'teachable', a special effort still needs to be made, and this will require appropriate training.

Physician interventions

The impact of brief advice by a physician is often underestimated. Although the absolute effect is relatively small, this is more than offset by the very large number of people who can be given such brief advice. There is growing evidence that this effect, although small, is significant and robust.

> The results of this review indicate the potential benefit from brief simple advice given by physicians to their smoking patients. The challenge as to whether or not this benefit will be realised depends on the extent to which physicians are prepared to systematically identify their smoking patients and offer them advice as a matter of routine.
>
> Providing follow-up, if possible, is likely to produce additional benefit. However, the marginal benefits of more intensive

interventions, including use of aids, is small and cannot be justified as a routine intervention in unselected smokers. They may, however, be of benefit for individual, motivated smokers. Nicotine replacement therapy [and Zyban] can improve quit rates irrespective of the intensity of advice offered, and should be considered an important adjunct to advice.

Silagy and Stead[11]

Pregnancy

One of the barriers to smoking cessation in pregnant women is the continued smoking of their partners. Some guidelines for promoting cessation in pregnant women are listed below.

- Encourage pregnant women to ask their partner to quit and/or provide a smoke-free home environment.
- Offer the woman's partner support and advice.
- Explain the impact of passive smoking on infants.
- Provide advice during teachable moments (e.g. immediately prior to ultrasound appointments).

There is substantial evidence that providing smoking cessation support in the maternity setting has significant benefits.

As smoking cessation programmes have been shown to increase smoking cessation, increase mean birth weight and reduce low birth weight, even if none of the effects is large, then smoking cessation programmes need to be implemented in all maternity care settings. Attention to smoking behaviour together with support for smoking cessation and relapse prevention needs to be as routine a part of antenatal care as the measurement of blood pressure. Local piloting of programmes shown elsewhere to be effective would be a good place to begin. In order to avoid 'victim-blaming', or the perception of victim-blaming, attention should be given to the consumer's concerns. Interventions involving additional group sessions during pregnancy have been reported as being extremely poorly attended in virtually all trials where they were planned, and it may be time to recommend that they be abandoned.

Given the clear difficulties which most women still smoking at the first antenatal visit have in stopping smoking, midwives,

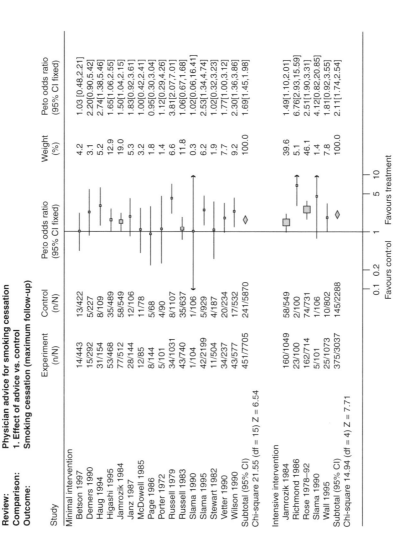

Figure 3.8: Findings with regard to physician advice for smoking cessation.[11]

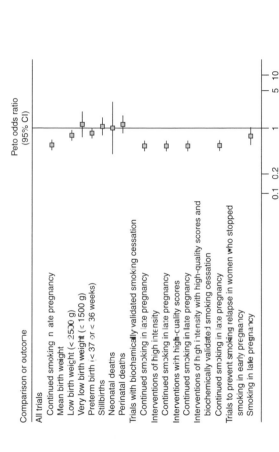

Figure 3.9: Findings with regard to interventions for promoting smoking cessation in pregnancy.[12]

general practitioners and obstetricians need to support strategies for smoking control in the whole community so as to reduce the initiation of smoking by young people: action to prevent sales of tobacco products to young people, prohibition of smoking in all public places, increases in tobacco taxation, workplace smoking cessation programmes and banning tobacco sponsorship of prestigious sporting and cultural events. Given the strong association between social inequality and continued smoking by pregnant women, and bearing in mind the contribution of smoking to the global burden of disease in developed market economies, midwives, general practitioners and obstetricians need to support strategies in the wider community to reduce social inequalities.

Lumley *et al.*[12]

Hospitalisation

Hospitalisation provides a teachable moment, especially if the reason for admission is related to smoking and the consequences of smoking. As well as providing a potential teachable moment, interventions that achieve either a reduction in smoking or complete cessation *prior* to a surgical intervention appear to reduce postoperative complications. Postoperative support also seems to be important, whether or not the surgery was elective.

The results support the use of smoking cessation interventions delivered during the hospitalisation period that also include follow-up for at least one month post-hospitalisation. Although such interventions were effective whether or not NRT was used, the results are compatible with data which show the effectiveness of NRT in other populations. There was no clear evidence that patients with different clinical diagnoses respond in different ways.

Rigotti *et al.*[13]

Role of GPs in the identification of teachable moments

One problem associated with the provision of brief advice in a primary care setting is the difficulty in providing such advice repetitively, as

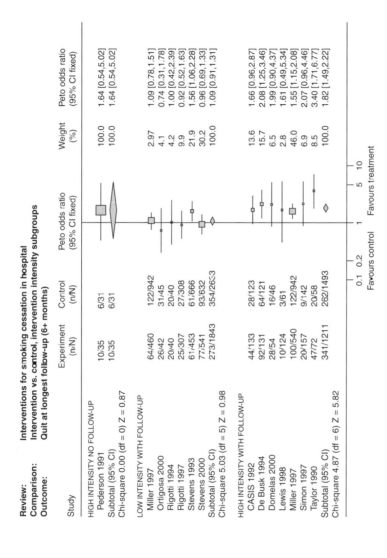

Figure 3.10: Findings with regard to interventions for smoking cessation in hospital settings.[13]

this may compromise the relationship with the patient. Therefore a potentially useful adjunct to such advice is the targeting of interventions towards individuals for whom a recent diagnosis provides the opportunity for a teachable moment.

> Primary care clinicians and policy makers should know that no intervention guarantees success, and several interventions are available that can improve prevention to some extent. Most well studied are group education and physician reminders, but other interventions (such as organisational interventions) are potentially useful as well.
>
> Hulscher et al.[14]

Combining with pharmacological interventions

Counselling by physicians and nurses, behavioural interventions (individual counselling or group therapy), nicotine replacement therapy and several pharmacological interventions (e.g. the antidepressants bupropion and nortriptyline) increase smoking cessation rates (see Chapter 4).

Accessibility of psychological and behavioural techniques

One problem with these techniques is that they require a high throughput if their provision is to be cost-effective. For example, group behavioural interventions are only likely to be practicable in a large metropolis where there is a sufficient population of smokers to provide a consistent throughput. The implementation of such interventions in smaller cities and rural areas is currently being piloted, and this has identified a need for flexibility with regard to both the frequency with which such programmes are run, and their location.

Alternative therapies

Acupuncture

Acupuncture has been used in the treatment of nicotine dependence in the West since an incidental observation was made in Hong Kong in the 1970s. Opium smokers who had been given electro-acupuncture for pain relief claimed that their opiate withdrawal symptoms were less severe than they had expected. Uncontrolled studies have suggested that acupuncture might also reduce the symptoms of nicotine withdrawal, and some remarkably high initial rates of success have been reported. For example, it has been claimed that 95% of 194 subjects were not smoking after three treatments in one week, falling to 34% after 12 months. An 88% success rate has also been reported in a large study of 514 subjects, but the long-term results were not stated. Clearly only randomised controlled studies can determine whether this is more than just a placebo effect.

> There is no evidence for the specific effectiveness of acupuncture in smoking cessation greater than a placebo effect
>
> White *et al.*[15]

Hypnotherapy

The rationale for hypnotherapy being a useful adjunct in smoking cessation is that, by acting on underlying impulses, it may weaken the desire to smoke, strengthen the will to stop, or improve the ability to focus on a treatment programme by increasing concentration. Many different hypnotherapy techniques have been employed, but the most frequently used approaches are variants of the 'one-session, three-point' method developed by Spiegel. This method attempts to modify patients' perceptions of smoking by using the potential of hypnotherapy to induce deep concentration. During the session the smoker is instructed that (1) smoking is a poison, (2) the body is entitled to protection from smoke and (3) there are advantages to life as a non-smoker. This approach also includes training in self-hypnosis, which may be as important as hypnosis by a therapist. Self-hypnosis can be used at will by the patient, and compliance rates may be higher and costs lower because only one session is required. In uncontrolled studies, six-month abstinence rates using this method have been reported to range from 20% to 35%.

> There is insufficient evidence to recommend hypnotherapy as a specific treatment for smoking cessation.
>
> Abbot *et al.*[16]

Summary of effective interventions

Table 3.1 Incremental effects of smoking cessation interventions on abstinence for 6 months or longer

Intervention	Target population	Quit rate[a]	Likely range of true quit rate[b]
Brief opportunistic advice from a physician to stop smoking	Smokers attending GP surgeries or outpatient clinics	2%	1–3%
Face-to-face intensive behavioural support from a specialist[c]	Moderate to heavy smokers seeking help with stopping	7%	3–10%
Face-to-face intensive behavioural support from a spccialist	Pregnant smokers	7%	5–9%
Face-to-face intensive behavioural support from a specialist[d]	Smokers admitted to hospital	4%	0–8%
Proactive telephone counselling[e]	Smokers wanting help with stopping, but not receiving face-to-face support	2%	1–4%
Written self-help materials	Smokers seeking help and not receiving other support	1%	0–2%
Nicotine gum	Moderate to heavy smokers receiving *limited* behavioural support[f]	5%	4–6%
Nicotine gum	Moderate to heavy smokers receiving *intensive* behavioural support	8%	6–10%

Table 3.1 Continued.

Intervention	Target population	Quit rate[a]	Likely range of true quit rate[b]
Nicotine transdermal patch	Moderate to heavy smokers receiving *limited* behavioural support	5%	4–7%
Nicotine transdermal patch	Moderate to heavy smokers receiving *intensive* behavioural support	6%	5–8%
Nicotine nasal spray	Moderate to heavy smokers receiving *intensive* behavioural support	12%	7–17%
Nicotine inhalator	Moderate to heavy smokers receiving *intensive* behavioural support	8%	4–12%
Nicotine sublingual tablet	Moderate to heavy smokers receiving *intensive* behavioural support	8%	1–14%
Bupropion (300 mg/day sustained release)	Moderate to heavy smokers receiving *intensive* behavioural support	9%	5–14%
Intensive behavioural support plus NRT or bupropion[g]	Moderate to heavy smokers seeking help from a smokers' clinic	13–19%	—

[a] Difference in > six-month abstinence rate between intervention and control/placebo in the studies reported; data are from Cochrane meta-analyses unless otherwise stated.

[b] The range within which one can be 95% confident that the true underlying value lies.

[c] Efficacy figures based on a subset of studies from the general population with biochemical verification.

[d] No Cochrane Review available; data from US Department of Health and Human Services (USDHHS) meta-analysis.

[e] No Cochrane Review available; data from USDHHS meta-analysis.

[f] The term 'limited behavioural support' refers to brief sessions required primarily for collecting data. Following the Cochrane definition, 'intensive behavioural support' was defined as an initial session lasting for more than 30 minutes, or an initial session lasting for less than 30 minutes plus more than two subsequent visits.

[g] Expected effect combining the effect of medication with the effect of behavioural support.

Summary of Cochrane Tobacco Addiction Group Reviews

1	Nicotine replacement therapy for smoking cessation	Silagy C, Mant D, Fowler G, Lancaster T
2	Physician advice for smoking cessation	Silagy C, Ketteridge S
3	Training health professionals in smoking cessation	Lancaster T, Silagy C, Fowler G, Spiers I
4	Acupuncture for smoking cessation	White AR, Rampes H
5	Clonidine for smoking cessation	Gourlay SG, Stead LF, Benowitz NL
6	Antidepressants for smoking cessation	Hughes JR, Stead LF, Lancaster TR
7	Anxiolytics for smoking cessation	Hughes JR, Stead LF, Lancaster TR
8	Lobeline for smoking cessation	Stead LF, Hughes JR
9	Silver acetate for smoking cessation	Lancaster T, Stead LF
10	Aversive smoking for smoking cessation	Hajek P, Stead LF
11	Mecamylamine for smoking cessation	Lancaster T, Stead LF
12	Hypnotherapy for smoking cessation	Abbot NC, Stead LF, White AR, Barnes J, Ernst E
13	Group behaviour therapy programmes for smoking cessation	Stead LF, Lancaster T
14	Mass media interventions for preventing smoking in young people	Sowden AJ, Arblaster L
15	Self-help interventions for smoking cessation	Lancaster T, Stead LF
16	Individual behavioural counselling for smoking cessation	Lancaster T, Stead LF
17	Nursing interventions for smoking cessation	Rice VH, Stead L
18	Interventions for preventing tobacco sales to minors	Lancaster T, Stead LF
19	Community interventions for preventing smoking in young people	Sowden AJ, Arblaster L
20	Interventions for preventing tobacco smoking in public places	Serra C, Cabezas C, Bonfill X, Pladevall-Vila M
21	Exercise interventions for smoking cessation	Ussher MH, West R, Taylor AH, McEwen A
22	Interventions for smoking cessation in hospitalised patients	Rigotti NA, Munafo MR, Murphy MFG, Stead LF
23	Telephone counselling for smoking cessation	Stead LF, Lancaster T
24	Opioid antagonists for smoking cessation	David S, Lancaster T, Stead LF
25	Interventions for preoperative smoking cessation	Moller A, Pederson T, Villebro N
26	Enhanced partner support to improve smoking cessation	Park EW, Schultz JK, Tudiver F, Campbell T, Becker L

Source: http://www.dphpc.ox.ac.uk/cochrane_tobacco/

Reflection exercise

Exercise 5

Having read through the material in this chapter, do you now have a good understanding of the range of psychological and behavioural techniques and how you can provide these for individuals who smoke, and when to refer patients to other professionals? You could look up the original references cited here or discuss the contents of the chapter with an appropriate colleague. Collate a list of sources of advice and help for patients in your locality.

> Now that you have completed this interactive reflection exercise, transfer the information to the empty template of the personal development plan on pages 169–178 if you are working on your own learning plan, or to the practice personal and professional development plan on pages 193–199 if you are working on a practice team learning plan. Don't forget to keep the evidence of your learning in your personal portfolio.

References

1 Butler C, Rollnick S, Cohen D, Russell I, Bachmann M and Stott N (1999) Motivational counselling versus brief advice for smokers in general practice: A randomised trial. *Br J Gen Pract.* **49**: 611–16.
2 Windsor RA, Lowe JB and Bartlett EE (1998) The effectiveness of a worksite self-help smoking cessation program: a randomized trial. *J Behav Med.* **11**: 407–21.
3 Lancaster T and Stead LF (2002) Individual behavioural counselling for smoking cessation (Cochrane Review). In: *The Cochrane Library, Issue 1.* Update Software, Oxford.
4 Hajek P and Stead LF (2002) Aversive smoking for smoking cessation (Cochrane Review). In: *The Cochrane Library, Issue 1.* Update Software, Oxford.
5 Ussher MH, West R, Taylor AH and McEwen A (2002) Exercise interventions for smoking cessation (Cochrane Review). In: *The Cochrane Library, Issue 1.* Update Software, Oxford.
6 Lancaster T and Stead LF (2002) Self-help interventions for smoking cessation (Cochrane Review). In: *The Cochrane Library, Issue 1.* Update Software, Oxford.

7 Stead LF and Lancaster T (2002) Telephone counselling for smoking cessation (Cochrane Review). In: *The Cochrane Library, Issue 1.* Update Software, Oxford.

8 Sowden A and Arblaster L (2002) Community interventions for preventing smoking in young people (Cochrane Review). In: *The Cochrane Library, Issue 1.* Update Software, Oxford.

9 Stead LF and Lancaster T (2002) Group behaviour therapy programmes for smoking cessation (Cochrane Review). In: *The Cochrane Library, Issue 1.* Update Software, Oxford.

10 Rice VH and Stead LF (2002) Nursing interventions for smoking cessation (Cochrane Review). In: *The Cochrane Library, Issue 1.* Update Software, Oxford.

11 Silagy C and Stead LF (2002) Physician advice for smoking cessation (Cochrane Review). In: *The Cochrane Library, Issue 1.* Update Software, Oxford.

12 Lumley J, Oliver S and Waters E (2002) Interventions for promoting smoking cessation during pregnancy (Cochrane Review). In: *The Cochrane Library, Issue 1.* Update Software, Oxford.

13 Rigotti NA, Munafo MR, Murphy MFG and Stead LF (2002) Interventions for smoking cessation in hospitalised patients (Cochrane Review). In: *The Cochrane Library, Issue 1.* Update Software, Oxford.

14 Hulscher MEJL, Wensing M, van der Weijden T and Grol R (2002) Interventions to implement prevention in primary care (Cochrane Review). In: *The Cochrane Library, Issue 1.* Update Software, Oxford.

15 White AR, Rampes H and Ernst E (2002) Acupuncture for smoking cessation (Cochrane Review). In: *The Cochrane Library, Issue 1.* Update Software, Oxford.

16 Abbot NC, Stead LF, White AR and Barnes J (2002) Hypnotherapy for smoking cessation (Cochrane Review). In: *The Cochrane Library, Issue 1.* Update Software, Oxford.

CHAPTER 4

Pharmacological interventions and new medications

> The cigarette is the syringe to deliver nicotine, but it is a dirty syringe.
>
> Professor Martin Jarvis,
> Report of the Scientific Committee on Tobacco and Health[1]

As described in the opening chapter, nicotine is a drug with a very strong addictive potential. Pharmacological interventions are common in the management of addiction, and nicotine is no exception to this. The most widely known and used pharmacological therapy for nicotine addiction is substitution therapy, more commonly known as nicotine replacement therapy (NRT). However, there are other pharmacological interventions, such as the recently licensed Zyban (bupropion/amfembutanone), which is an atypical antidepressant. Other novel interventions are also currently being trialled for their efficacy, although some of them are hampered by their side-effect profile.

Although pharmacological interventions such as NRT and Zyban have been shown to increase the likelihood of successfully stopping smoking, the efficacy of these interventions can be increased by (and may depend on) combining them with psychological and behavioural techniques (described in more detail in Chapter 3). It is worth bearing in mind that the two approaches are highly complementary.

Nicotine replacement therapy (NRT)

Rationale for use

Substitution therapy is based on a model of cigarette smoking which suggests that the withdrawal syndrome (see below) is a consequence of nicotine deprivation once dependence on the drug has become established in the smoker. Therefore, by replacing some of the nicotine that is normally taken in while smoking, while continuing to abstain from smoking, the withdrawal effects can be reduced, thereby increasing the likelihood of successfully stopping smoking. It is by far the most widely known and used pharmacological intervention for nicotine dependence, and its efficacy is now well established. However, it is not clear precisely how NRT works. Even the most rapidly delivered nicotine replacement does not mimic the arterial spike produced by smoking a cigarette, which provides much of the reinforcing and addictive potential of cigarette smoking. Nevertheless, the venous levels of nicotine are approximately 50% of those achieved during moderately heavy smoking, and appear to offer some relief.

Research is in progress to determine whether the replacement level can be improved by using stronger doses of NRT or combined modalities, but this practice is not currently recommended in the product licences.

The withdrawal syndrome is characterised by the symptoms listed in Table 4.1.

In addition, there are several signs associated with smoking cessation (*see* Chapter 2). For example, most smokers (around 80%) gain weight

Table 4.1 Symptoms of nicotine withdrawal syndrome

Withdrawal symptom	Duration	Proportion affected
Irritability or aggression	< 4 weeks	50%
Depression	< 4 weeks	60%
Restlessness	< 4 weeks	60%
Poor concentration	< 2 weeks	60%
Increased appetite	> 10 weeks	70%
Light-headedness	< 48 hours	10%
Sleep disturbance	< 1 week	25%
Mouth ulcers	< 4 weeks	50%
Craving	> 2 weeks	70%

Source: Action on Smoking and Health.[2]

once they stop smoking (primarily as a consequence of the increased appetite experienced on stopping), although the weight gain in the long term is usually minor. This is a source of concern for many, but it is important to emphasise that:

- the health risks of weight gain are far outweighed by the health benefits of stopping smoking
- dieting should not be attempted in parallel with the attempt to stop smoking.

Any attempt to stop smoking is difficult enough on its own without the added pressure of attempting to diet successfully as well.

Withdrawal-oriented therapy is therefore based on the notion that smokers who wish to stop but who find this difficult are addicted to nicotine, and that nicotine deprivation is the main remediable source of difficulty in stopping.

Types of NRT

Nicotine chewing gum was developed in the late 1960s, for use by those in situations where they were prevented from smoking (e.g. sub-mariners in enclosed spaces). It has been available for clinical use since the early 1980s, and has been rigorously evaluated in terms of its clinical efficacy and safety. Other types of NRT have subsequently been developed, and are described below. Since the intervention is designed to support a behavioural change, rather than to treat illness, it requires different advice and explanation ('psychological packaging') to more commonly prescribed drugs.

Typical NRT products include the following:

- NRT gum (low strength)
- NRT gum (high strength)
- NRT patch (of varying strengths, tapering doses and both 16- and 24-hour delivery periods)
- NRT inhalator
- NRT sublingual tablet
- NRT lozenge
- NRT nasal spray.

The principal differences between these various delivery devices lie in the speed of uptake of nicotine and the period of time over which nicotine is released. For example, NRT patches release a steady dose of nicotine over the course of the day (usually a 16-hour period, but also available for delivery over a 24-hour period). Sublingual tablets and lozenges also release a steady dose of nicotine, but over a shorter period. The other delivery devices (gum, inhaler and nasal spray) all allow the delivery of nicotine on demand in order to satisfy periodic increases in craving (although the term 'inhalator' is misleading, as most absorption takes place in the buccal mucosa). The NRT nasal spray is only available on prescription, mainly due to the speed of uptake of nicotine by this means, which has led to concerns about its addictive potential. All of the other forms are available in pharmacies over the counter, while gum has a general sales licence and is available in supermarkets.

The overall efficacy of these products does not differ widely. NRT gum has been shown to be maximally effective as part of a smoking cessation package that includes psychological or group support. However, GPs who have been briefed in its use also appear to obtain better results. The NRT patch has recently been shown to be effective in a GP setting, possibly because of greater patient compliance in this context than with NRT gum, although it may be because its use is more quickly and readily explained than the use of NRT gum.

One issue that is currently being investigated is the potential for NRT combination therapy (e.g. combining the slow and constant release of nicotine by means of an NRT patch and another delivery device that offers rapid, controllable titration of the nicotine dose by the patient, such as an NRT inhaler or NRT gum). However, the terms of the product licences for the different forms currently advise against this.

Evidence for the efficacy of NRT

A recent review of 108 clinical trials of the effectiveness of all types of NRT, published in the Cochrane Library,[3] reached the following conclusions:

1   All of the commercially available forms of NRT (nicotine gum, nicotine transdermal patch, nicotine nasal spray, nicotine inhalator and nicotine sublingual tablet) are effective as part of a strategy to promote smoking cessation. They increase long-term quit rates by approximately 1.5- to twofold regardless of the setting. The use of NRT should be preferentially targeted at smokers who are motivated to quit (as demonstrated by their initiative in requesting assistance) and who have high levels of nicotine dependency. There is little evidence for the role of NRT in individuals who smoke less

than 10–15 cigarettes per day (although there is no reason why it should *not* work).

2   The choice of which form to use should reflect patient needs, preferences, tolerability and cost considerations. Patches are likely to be easier to use than gum or nasal spray in primary care settings.

3   Eight weeks of patch therapy is as effective as longer courses, and there is no evidence that tapered therapy is better than abrupt withdrawal. Wearing the patch only during waking hours (16 hours a day) is as effective as wearing it for 24 hours a day, but a patch of appropriate strength should be used.

4   If gum is used, it may be offered on a fixed-dose or ad-lib basis. For highly dependent smokers, or those who have failed with 2 mg gum, 4 mg gum should be offered.

5   There is some evidence of a small benefit from combining the nicotine patch with a form that allows ad-lib dosing compared with the use of a single form. Use of combination therapy may be considered for patients who have been unable to quit using a single type of NRT.

6   There is borderline evidence that a small benefit is obtained from use of the nicotine patch at doses higher than 22 mg/24 hours or 15 mg/16 hours, compared with standard-dose patches. Use of these higher doses may be considered for heavy smokers (>30 cigarettes a day), or for patients who are relapsing because of persistent craving and withdrawal symptoms on standard-dose therapy.

7   The effectiveness of NRT appears to be largely independent of the intensity of additional support provided for the smoker. Since all of the trials of NRT reported to date have included at least some form of brief advice to the smoker, this represents the minimum that should be offered in order to ensure its effectiveness. Provision of more intense levels of support, although beneficial in increasing the likelihood of quitting, is not essential to the success of NRT.

8   There is minimal evidence that a repeated course of NRT in patients who have relapsed after recent use of nicotine patches will result in a small additional probability of quitting.

9   NRT does not lead to an increased risk of adverse cardiovascular events in smokers with a history of cardiovascular disease.

10 Nicotine patches were found to be less effective than bupropion (*see* below) in one trial. However, any decision about which pharmacotherapies to use should take into account potential adverse effects as well as benefits.

11 Finally, marketing claims by manufacturers of NRT products should reflect these points and avoid the possible misunderstanding by

health professionals and members of the public that any of these products alone offers a magical 'cure' for the smoking habit.

Novel delivery systems

Alternative delivery systems

Table 4.2 summarises the results of several clinical trials of the effectiveness of alternative nicotine replacement therapy delivery systems.

Table 4.2 Effectiveness of alternative nicotine replacement therapy delivery systems

Type of NRT	Number of trials	Number/ total	Percentage	Number/ total	Percentage	Numbers needed to treat (95% CI)
		Patients stopped smoking at 6–12 months				
All trials						
Gum	48	1453/7387	20	1084/9319	12	12 (11–14)
Patch	31	1384/9708	14	495/5969	8	17 (14–20)
Intranasal spray	4	107/448	24	52/439	12	8 (6–14)
Inhalator	4	84/490	14	44/486	8	12 (8–26)
Sublingual tablet	2	49/243	20	31/245	13	13 (7–103)
Large trials[a]						
Gum	18	792/5126	15	710/7308	10	17 (14–22)
Patch	14	1115/8333	13	352/4615	8	17 (15–21)
Cessation rate with control < 10%						
Gum	15	299/3370	9	315/5192	6	36 (25–61)
Patch	17	482/4219	11	193/3440	6	17 (14–22)

[a] Large trials were those with more than 250 participants in NRT and placebo groups combined.
Source: *Bandolier.*[4]

Cost of NRT

Cost per life-year saved

In a recent review, the cost per life-year saved for smoking cessation interventions ranged from £344 to £785 depending on the intensity of the intervention and the age of the patient. When assessed against a wide range of life-saving interventions, this compares very favourably.

Raw *et al.*[5] assessed the cost per life-year saved of different primary care interventions as follows:

- brief GP advice; £112
- brief GP advice + leaflet; £142
- brief GP advice + leaflet + NRT; £173
- brief GP advice + leaflet + NRT + specialist cessation service; £160.

Although such calculations are complex, resulting in slight disparities in the results, this compares extremely favourably with other interventions. For example, the National Institute for Clinical Excellence (NICE) uses a benchmark cost-effectiveness figure of £30 000 per life-year saved in its health technology assessments for acceptability for NHS expenditure.[6] Therefore the figures for smoking cessation intervention even when the higher estimates are used, suggest a cost-effectiveness that is 40–50 times better than the NICE threshold.

One example serves to illustrate the cost-effectiveness of smoking cessation interventions. Over 80% of patients who are prescribed statins would fall below the risk threshold for these drugs if they stopped smoking, and 87% of those who are prescribed statins *are* smokers. The cost-effectiveness of statins is one-thirteenth that of smoking cessation interventions, while ten times more will be spent on statins in one year than on smoking cessation.

Cost relative to smoking

The cost of NRT to the patient is approximately equal to the cost of smoking, but this assumes a successful cessation attempt. The availability of NRT on prescription should go some way towards removing this particularly salient barrier to the use of NRT.

On average, the cost of NRT is approximately £10 to £20 per week, compared to about £25 per week to support a '20-a-day' habit.

Further information from the Department of Health on NRT on prescription can be found at http://www.doh.gov.uk/nrt/.

Barriers to use

Research has also identified potential barriers to the use of smoking cessation therapies, in particular NRT, including reduced awareness as a result of decreasing advertising, market fatigue with more established therapies, concerns about the safety and cost of treatments, and a lack of knowledge of the availability of NRT on prescription. In general, however, NRT is widely regarded as acceptable and benign, the principal barrier to its use being a financial one. Other potential barriers include a lack of knowledge of the effectiveness of NRT, which suggests a possible role for the GP in providing information about it.

Withdrawal and side-effects

Withdrawal from nicotine replacement therapy

Some patients express concern that they will become addicted to NRT, but this is very rare, primarily because the dosage of nicotine and the speed of uptake into the arterial circulation are both far less than when nicotine is delivered by cigarette. Studies have shown that it is much easier to give up the patch than it would be to give up cigarettes, for two reasons. First, people usually develop cravings for things that provide immediate satisfaction. With NRT, the nicotine level in the body remains relatively constant day after day, and does not mimic the nicotine delivery from a cigarette. There is not immediate satisfaction, so there is little craving for a patch (one exception to this is NRT nasal spray, which provides the fastest delivery of nicotine of any form of NRT – hence its availability only on prescription). Secondly, anything that people do often, such as smoking, becomes a habit. However, since NRT is generally used less frequently, there is no strong habit to break.

Most importantly, the concern that NRT may be addictive can lead to its under-use, which severely reduces its effectiveness in aiding any cessation attempt.

Side-effects

There are several side-effects associated with the use of NRT, but in general most side-effects are not serious. Nicotine gum can cause jaw-muscle ache and damage dental work (i.e. fillings and dentures). If it is chewed too fast, nicotine gum can cause light-headedness, hiccups, heart palpitations and stomach upset. Known side-effects include the following:

- headaches
- dizziness

- upset stomach
- weakness
- blurred vision
- vivid dreams and insomnia (especially if a 24-hour patch is used)
- mild itching and burning on the skin (in the case of the patch)
- diarrhoea.

It is important to distinguish side-effects from withdrawal symptoms in NRT users who quit, since misinterpretation of these by the quitter can lead to concern.

There is also current debate as to whether NRT is safe for use by pregnant women and individuals with existing heart disease, although it is certainly true that continued smoking is far more harmful in both cases than the use of NRT. Most NRT users take in less nicotine (and no other harmful substances) when using any NRT product and abstaining from smoking, compared with when they are smoking normally. The use of a 16-hour patch of NRT during the daytime also means that they are absorbing nicotine in a similar pattern over time to when they are smoking. It is difficult to see how this could be *more* harmful than smoking, provided that smokers are instructed not to smoke and use NRT at the same time.

A recent Action on Smoking and Health (ASH) position statement concluded:

> We would like to register concern about the continued requirement to display a warning to discourage pregnant women from using NRT products. Even the most intensive use of NRT during pregnancy could not remotely match the dangers to mother or child of continued smoking. By discouraging pregnant women from using NRT products to stop smoking, there are without doubt women smoking through pregnancy who would have successfully quit with the aid of NRT products. This far greater harm should be weighed against the small net impact associated with NRT use by pregnant women who would have been able to quit without it.

Advising on NRT use

Any smoker who is considering making a cessation attempt should be advised to use NRT unless this is specifically contraindicated.

NRT products vary in the following respects:

- speed of delivery
- dose delivered
- time over which nicotine is absorbed
- ease of use
- frequency of use
- side-effects
- behavioural replacement (hand/mouth).

NRT should be recommended if:

- prior cessation attempts have failed
- prior cessation attempts have resulted in strong withdrawal symptoms
- dependence is high (e.g. the patient smokes a cigarette soon after waking, *not* necessarily a high number of cigarettes per day)
- expectations of success are low.

Patients should be informed of the following:

- rationale for use (nicotine as an addictive substance)
- the best way to use NRT (including how much, and for how long)
- side-effects
- the need to set a quit date and stop completely, rather than cut down gradually.

The following may reduce the likelihood of success:

- unrealistic expectations
- incorrect use (using too little, using it irregularly or stopping too early)
- smoking while using NRT.

There is substantial evidence that cutting down gradually reduces the likelihood of successful cessation. In addition, smoking fewer cigarettes carries minimal health benefits, as smokers modify their smoking behaviour so as to extract the same dose of nicotine (and many toxins) from fewer cigarettes (e.g. by inhaling for longer). For the same reason, there is little benefit in switching to lower-tar brands.

In addition, it should be made clear that NRT is not a simple cure for nicotine addiction, and that will-power and a desire to succeed are also crucial. NRT helps to alleviate some of the initial withdrawal symptoms, but the second stage of any cessation attempt involves maintaining abstinence after the initial four-week period of withdrawal has passed. Moreover, NRT does not completely remove the withdrawal

Table 4.3 Characteristics of different types of NRT

Patch	Gum	Inhalator	Lozenge/ microtab	Nasal spray
Use one patch daily; 16-hour or 24-hour versions; minimal side-effects	Use as frequently as one would use cigarettes; needs to be used correctly; taste is initially aversive	Puff for 20 minutes hourly; lasts for 3×20 minutes; replaces habit/ behaviour	Dissolves under tongue; use 15–30 tablets daily; some local irritation occurs initially	Spray into nostril hourly; only available on prescription; initially very aversive

symptoms associated with cessation, and it provides less satisfaction (due to a lower dose and slower release) than cigarettes.

Other medications

Antidepressants

The value of bupropion (Zyban) was first recognised in the USA when it was used as an (atypical) antidepressant. A large number of anecdotal reports from those using the drug suggested that cravings following smoking cessation were reduced in those taking bupropion. The main contraindication to its use is an elevated risk of seizures; the risk of seizures is estimated to be about 1 in 1000. Reducing the seizure risk by not prescribing the drug to patients with the relevant contraindications reduces the number who might benefit from it substantially.

> The early results for several antidepressants, especially bupropion, are sufficient to endorse their use in medical practice. Nicotine replacement therapy has proven efficacy in over 80 studies . . . and has a very benign side-effect profile. Bupropion is now recommended for first-line pharmacotherapy alongside nicotine replacement therapy, in the updated US clinical practice guideline . . . . There is insufficient published evidence to recommend bupropion in preference to NRT or vice versa. Smokers with a previous history of depression or mild current depression have not been

shown to do better with antidepressants than NRT. Patient preferences, cost, availability and side-effect profile will all need to be taken into account. Bupropion may also be helpful in those who fail nicotine replacement. Nortriptyline may be considered a second-line therapy as it has more side-effects . . . Slow-release bupropion, under the name Zyban, is licensed for smoking cessation in North America and the European Union, but is not available in many other countries. However, under the name Wellbutrin SR it is licensed for depression in other countries.

More research is needed with different antidepressants to determine better which antidepressants or classes of antidepressants are effective in smoking cessation. Determining this could provide insight into the biological factors controlling nicotine dependence and smoking. For example, if only antidepressants with noradrenergic effects (which is true for bupropion and nortriptyline) were effective, it would suggest this system, rather than dopamine (which is affected substantially by bupropion but not by nortriptyline) alone, is important in nicotine dependence. The use of antidepressants in combination with nicotine replacement therapy also needs to be further investigated. Head-to-head trials are needed to compare the antidepressant therapies with nicotine replacement, to establish equivalence of efficacy. Trials also need to assess not only efficacy but acceptability, compliance and side-effects to better approximate effectiveness. Trials are also needed in which NRT is used as an active initial therapy and 'failures' are randomly allocated to antidepressants or placebo.

Hughes *et al.*[7]

Clive Bates, the director of Action on Smoking and Health (ASH), reports as follows:

Zyban is an effective anti-smoking treatment, and . . . the first studies show very promising success rates. But until more studies have been done, it is too soon to be making comparisons between NRT and Zyban. Both products have an important role to play and will meet smokers' needs in different ways. The products may also be most effective when used in combination.[2]

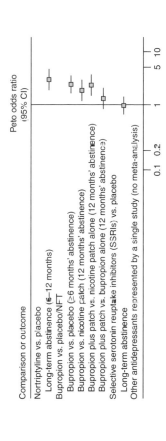

Figure 4.1: Findings with regard to antidepressant interventions for smoking cessation.[7]

Anxiolytics

Given that subjective increases in anxiety, tension and restlessness constitute an important part of the withdrawal syndrome, this would suggest that pharmacological interventions which ameliorate these symptoms should be effective in supporting a cessation attempt. There is some evidence that clonidine may be effective, but its side-effect profile may limit its use.

> The available evidence neither supports nor rules out an effect of anxiolytics on smoking cessation. In view of this uncertainty and the side-effects of the drugs, there is little justification for using them. One drug with some anxiolytic effects, clonidine, does show evidence of efficacy . . . but the incidence of side-effects from clonidine is relatively high.
>
> Hughes *et al.*[8]

> On the basis of available studies it is reasonable to consider oral or transdermal clonidine as a second-line pharmacotherapy for smoking cessation. Close medical supervision is essential to titrate the dose appropriately and monitor for potentially severe adverse effects. The increasing use of antidepressants as an alternative, or complement, to nicotine replacement means that clonidine is unlikely to be used in primary care settings, but may play some role in specialist treatment.
>
> The finding that clonidine, an alpha-2-adrenergic and imidazoline receptor agonist, has efficacy in smoking cessation suggests that further work in this area is warranted. A key aspect of future research will be whether the efficacy of drugs acting via these mechanisms can be dissociated from adverse effects. Such improvements in the benefit/risk ratio might allow first-line use in a broad population of smokers.
>
> Gourlay *et al.*[9]

Lobeline

Lobeline is an alkaloid derived from the leaves of an Indian tobacco plant, *Lobelia inflata*. It was first synthesised in the early 1900s and

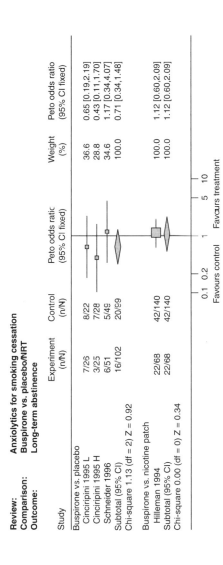

Figure 4.2: Findings with regard to anxiolytic interventions for smoking cessation.[8]

was classified as a partial nicotinic agonist. Its first reported use in aiding smoking cessation was in the 1930s. Unfortunately, there is insufficient evidence to allow its efficacy in smoking cessation to be assessed.

There are no well-conducted trials with long-term follow-up. There is therefore no evidence that lobeline can aid smoking cessation.

Stead and Hughes[10]

Mecamylamine

Mecamylamine is a nicotinic acetylcholinergic-receptor antagonist. Two published studies have provided evidence for the efficacy of mecamylamine as an intervention for smoking cessation.

In the absence of evidence of a sustained effect on quitting from large-scale studies, it is premature to recommend the addition of mecamylamine to nicotine replacement for smoking cessation. However, existing research suggests that, used in low dose, mecamylamine can be tolerated, and that there is preliminary evidence to suggest that it may be a useful additional agent in smoking cessation, particularly in combination with nicotine replacement.

Further large-scale studies are required to determine whether mecamylamine, combined with nicotine replacement, is more effective than nicotine alone. In addition, a number of questions remain to be answered about the best dose and timing if this therapy is used. In particular, questions remain about whether mecamylamine is more effective when given prior to, or following, cessation, and how it is best combined with nicotine replacement. Studies using a transdermal patch delivering both nicotine and mecamylamine are reported to be in progress.

Lancaster and Stead[11]

Opioid antagonists

As their name suggests, these drugs (e.g. naloxone and naltrexone) are opioid-receptor antagonists. In addition to evidence which suggests a possible reinforcing role for the endogenous opioid system in smoking, findings from other studies suggest that this system might be involved in mediating nicotine withdrawal. Studies have shown that the opioid antagonist naloxone precipitates nicotine withdrawal in nicotine-maintained rats, and nicotine-induced reversal of this withdrawal syndrome is antagonised by naloxone.

There is no evidence at present to support the clinical use of naltrexone or other opioid antagonists for smoking cessation.

More research is needed with larger sample sizes to determine whether naltrexone is efficacious for smoking cessation. Determining this would allow clinicians either to consider naltrexone as a second-line medication for smoking cessation, or to exclude naltrexone from our current armamentarium of smoking cessation medications. Research is also needed to investigate the efficacy of combining naltrexone with other smoking cessation medications that appear to diminish withdrawal symptoms and negative affect (e.g. bupropion, nortriptyline, clonidine, etc.).

David et al.[12]

Silver acetate

The rationale for the use of silver acetate is that it alters the *taste* of cigarette smoking adversely. Unfortunately, the evidence for its efficacy in supporting smoking cessation is not promising.

Although a possible small effect of silver acetate in promoting smoking cessation has not been disproved, any such effect is likely to be very small, and less than that proven for nicotine replacement therapy. There is therefore little role for silver acetate for promoting smoking cessation in the clinical setting.

Further research on silver acetate for smoking cessation is unlikely to be helpful.

Lancaster and Stead[13]

Combination treatment

Although few studies have been reported, there is an excellent rationale for using combined therapies for nicotine dependence, especially when a slow-delivery form of NRT (patch) or other pharmacological therapy is combined with a more rapid delivery system (nicotine gum or nicotine nasal spray). Nicotine gum in combination with nicotine patch therapy has been shown to reduce withdrawal symptoms more effectively than either medication alone. Furthermore, when used in combination, the nicotine patch and nicotine gum produce significantly higher abstinence rates compared with nicotine gum alone. In addition, a single 1-mg dose of nicotine nasal spray was shown to provide more immediate relief of craving for a cigarette than a single 4-mg dose of nicotine gum. These findings provide a basis for the 'as-needed' use of nicotine nasal spray to control withdrawal symptoms, in combination with other medications with longer-acting effects.

In a patch–bupropion trial, bupropion SR 300 mg daily was used in combination with a 21-mg nicotine patch. All three active treatment groups were more effective than placebo, and bupropion SR was associated with significantly higher cessation rates compared with the nicotine patch. Although the combination of bupropion SR and the nicotine patch produced the highest smoking cessation rates, this was not significantly different to bupropion SR alone ($P = 0.06$). Nonetheless, because NRT and bupropion act in different ways and on different parts of the brain, the combination of the two therapies makes pharmacological sense.

Furthermore, the use of higher doses of nicotine patch therapy (i.e. more than one patch at a time) may be appropriate for some more strongly addicted smokers, especially heavy smokers (2 packs/ day), since they will be significantly under-dosed if they use single-dose patch therapy. High-dose therapy can also be used in smokers who previously failed single-dose therapy because their nicotine withdrawal symptoms were not adequately relieved. High-dose therapy has been shown to be safe and tolerable in individuals who smoked 20 or more cigarettes per day. To date, no trials have reported using more than two pharmacological agents at one time. However, in clinical practice as many as four pharmacotherapies (three NRTs plus bupropion) have been used simultaneously in patients with severe nicotine dependence in an inpatient treatment programme.

Reflection exercises

Exercise 6

Review the extent to which you are successful in helping patients who smoke to quit and to remain ex-smokers. Look at the quit rates of people attending any smoking cessation services that you provide, at three months after the initial consultation and at 6 or 12 month follow-up. What do you and your team need to learn from the results of this exercise? What reorganisation of the services that you provide in the practice could you make?

Exercise 7

Invite the local community pharmacist who is engaged in 'stopping people smoking' initiatives to join you in your practice for an educational session. Invite them to contribute to the review of a relevant practice protocol, or to take part in a general discussion of your learning needs as a practice. You could feed back comments from patients about your practice services or your prescribing of pharmacological interventions (such as those described in this chapter).

Exercise 8

Undertake a significant event audit of an adverse incident that has occurred in connection with an intervention for smoking cessation (e.g. a patient with established coronary heart disease and/or diabetes who has resumed smoking again after three months without smoking cigarettes). You could use the same approach to review the prescribing of a medication for a patient in whom it was contra-indicated. Look at the circumstances leading up to the event. Undertake the significant event audit by yourself or, better still, with a colleague or your team.

If you are unsure how to undertake a significant event audit, the method is well described in Wakley G, Chambers R and Field S (2000) *Continuing Professional Development in Primary Care: making it happen.* Radcliffe Medical Press, Oxford.

Now that you have completed this interactive reflection exercise, transfer the information to the empty template of the personal development plan on pages 169–178 if you are working on your own learning plan, or to the practice personal and professional development plan on pages 193–199 if you are working on a practice team learning plan. Don't forget to keep the evidence of your learning in your personal portfolio.

References

1 Department of Health (1998) *Report of the Scientific Committee on Tobacco and Health.* The Stationery Office, London.
2 Action on Smoking and Health (2002) http://www.ash.org.uk/.
3 Silagy C, Lancaster T, Stead L, Mant D and Fowler G (2002) Nicotine replacement therapy for smoking cessation (Cochrane Review). In: *The Cochrane Library, Issue 1.* Update Software, Oxford.
4 *Bandolier.* http://www.jr2.ox.ac.uk/bandolier/.
5 Raw M, McNeill A and West R (1998) Smoking cessation guidelines for health professionals. A guide to effective smoking cessation interventions for the healthcare system. *Thorax.* **53** (**Supplement 5**): S11–19.
6 Stapleton JR (2001) *Cost-Effectiveness of NHS Smoking Cessation Services.* Action on Smoking and Health. http://www.ash.org.uk/html/cessation/ashcost.pdf.
7 Hughes JR, Stead LF and Lancaster T (2002) Antidepressants for smoking cessation (Cochrane Review). In: *The Cochrane Library, Issue 1.* Update Software, Oxford.
8 Hughes JR, Stead LF and Lancaster T (2002) Anxiolytics for smoking cessation (Cochrane Review). In: *The Cochrane Library, Issue 1.* Update Software, Oxford.
9 Gourlay SG, Stead LF and Benowitz NL (2002) Clonidine for smoking cessation (Cochrane Review). In: *The Cochrane Library, Issue 1.* Update Software, Oxford.
10 Stead LF and Hughes JR (2002) Lobeline for smoking cessation (Cochrane Review). In: *The Cochrane Library, Issue 1.* Update Software, Oxford.
11 Lancaster T and Stead LF (2002) Mecamylamine (a nicotine antagonist) for smoking cessation (Cochrane Review). In: *The Cochrane Library, Issue 1.* Update Software, Oxford.
12 David S, Lancaster T and Stead LF (2002) Opioid antagonists for smoking cessation (Cochrane Review). In: *The Cochrane Library, Issue 1.* Update Software, Oxford.
13 Lancaster T and Stead LF (2002) Silver acetate for smoking cessation (Cochrane Review). In: *The Cochrane Library, Issue 1.* Update Software, Oxford.

CHAPTER 5

Practice policies and attitudes

Despite ties of family and history, the consequences of cultivating the potato and the tobacco plant could hardly be more divergent.

> According to Huron Indian myth, when the land was barren and the people were starving, the Great Spirit sent a woman to save humanity. As she travelled over the world, everywhere her right hand touched the soil there grew potatoes, and where her left hand touched there grew corn. When the world was rich and fertile, she sat down and rested. When she arose, there grew tobacco.

In South America, the Spanish Conquistadors failed in their search for El Dorado but found the potato (first recorded in 1553 by Pedro Cieza de Leon, in his journal *Chronicle of Peru*). Its cultivation has led to it becoming a staple food for the world.

In North America, Indians presented Columbus with the gift of tobacco (botanical sibling of the potato) in 1492. If current world smoking patterns persist, its cultivation will be the cause of death of a half a billion of the world's population alive today.

Attitudes to tobacco have changed. In 1566, Catherine de Medici, Queen of France, was so impressed by the effect of snuff on her migraine that she decreed tobacco should be termed Herba Regina. Nearly 500 years later it is the single largest avoidable cause of deaths, admissions to hospital and GP consultations in the UK. Cigarette smoking in 1997–98 caused an estimated 480 000 patients to consult their GPs for ischaemic heart disease, 20 000 to consult them for stroke and 600 000 for chronic obstructive pulmonary disease.

As the effects of smoking on public health have become more evident, policy initiatives in the UK have in general become correspondingly more enlightened. However, only recently have GPs been provided with the 'full set of tools' necessary to offer effective

interventions for nicotine addiction. Beyond a basic contractual obliga-
tion to offer advice opportunistically, there was no incentive for GPs to
do more until the 1990 Health Promotion contract, when reimbursement was made available. In 1996, that contract was replaced by a
looser structure, which required GPs to produce a description of their
proposed health promotion activities for approval, but which did not
define smoking cessation as a required activity. It was only at the turn
of the century that GPs were given the option of prescribing on the NHS
effective drugs that would help smokers to quit.

The White Paper entitled 'Smoking Kills', which was published in
December 1998, was an acknowledgement of the protean consequences
of smoking.[1] The tobacco strategy set out a comprehensive plan of
action, backed by more than £100 million over the succeeding three
years. It has attempted to cover the following areas:

- action to protect children and young people
- setting up a nationwide specialist smoking cessation service
- ending tobacco advertising and sponsorship
- an anti-smoking advertising campaign
- action on tobacco smuggling
- measures to reduce passive smoking at work.

The targets for England (there are separate targets for Wales and Scot-
land) are to reduce smoking rates in the following three areas:

1 *children*: from rates of 13% for 11- to 15-year-olds in 1996 to 9% by
   2010 (11% by 2005)
2 *adults*: from 28% in 1996 to 24% by 2010 (26% by 2005)
3 *women smoking in pregnancy*: from 23% in 1995 to 15% by 2010
   (18% by 2005).

In order to meet the targets set out in the paper, the requirement for a
co-ordinated anti-smoking strategy that 'joins up' activities in diverse
organisations at national and local levels was acknowledged. A total of
14 government and supra-national organisations are cited as being
instrumental in implementing the policy.

Integration at a local level, across all fields of healthcare, in education, in places of work and public areas, is arguably even more
important for achieving these targets. Guidelines for UK primary
care[2] were published in 1998, but general practice will need not only
to demonstrate a culture that is sympathetic to smoking prevention and
cessation, but also to link activities to local initiatives and with the
efforts of other concerned groups.

Smoking cessation work is increasingly – and appropriately –
undertaken in a variety of other settings by, for example, pharmacists,

dentists and teachers. Templates for audit and accepted quality standards in these types of areas are becoming increasingly available. The effectiveness of the tobacco strategy overall, and in primary care in particular, has much to gain from sharing experience, knowledge and resources.

For example, the Royal Pharmaceutical Society of Great Britain (RPSGB) has recommended that all pharmacists and counter staff should undergo appropriate training in smoking cessation and communication skills. The roles of the pharmacist in smoking cessation are not confined to simply giving advice about medication, but also include the following:

- encouraging smokers to voice their concerns about smoking
- encouraging smokers to make their own decisions about the need for change
- supplying information to the smoker to help them to make an informed choice
- exploring with the smoker the benefits and disadvantages of quitting
- providing a detailed plan of how to make the change
- helping with the implementation of the quitting strategy
- helping the person to remain a non-smoker.

The RPSGB has developed audit templates and helped to establish standards that can be adapted at local level.

Inter-referral, linking data recording and co-ordinated local campaigns all present opportunities to minimise effort and maximise effect.

Specialist smoking cessation services

A key part of the strategy defined in the 1998 White Paper was the setting up of a specialist smoking cessation service. In the first year (1999–2000), £10 million were allocated to Health Action Zones to begin the process. Access to specialist services is now available throughout the UK.

The specialist smoking cessation service has a role in care, through midwifery services, pharmacists, dental services and other healthcare settings. In addition to the brief advice that is offered to all smokers in these settings, it also includes provision of specialist services to smokers who need intensive support for their attempt to quit the habit.

The two core functions of the specialist service are training and support for professionals, and the provision of specialist smoking cessation advice to smokers.

Training is offered to primary and secondary care teams at two levels:

- *level 1*: training in brief interventions for primary healthcare teams, dentists, pharmacists, specialist nurses and community professionals
- *level 2*: training for intermediate Smoking Cessation Advisers in primary healthcare teams, cardiac rehabilitation teams, community midwifery services, specialist nurses and other community-based healthcare professionals. Additional training in specific topics to support these professionals is available, including the use of nicotine replacement therapy, monitoring procedures, raising the issue of smoking with clients, and training for professionals who want to run groups for stopping smoking.

In primary care, a key educational aim is to develop the role of a smoking cessation adviser for each practice, which could be taken on by a GP, practice nurse or health visitor, for example. Regular educational updates for advisers are provided by the service, and the role includes cascading this information down to other members of the primary healthcare team.

Examples of the support that is available to primary care may vary between areas, but can include any of the following:

- setting up and maintaining a practice smoking cessation clinic
- providing literature and online support for smokers
- advice and support with regard to entering smoking cessation data in practice computer systems
- provision of carbon monoxide monitors
- updating the primary healthcare team about developments in smoking cessation.

Many primary healthcare teams in England now have at least one trained Smoking Cessation Adviser. For example, in Oxfordshire there are now over 170 such advisers, including some in secondary care and non-health settings.

The cost-effectiveness of the NHS smoking cessation service to date has recently been assessed as being up to £800 per life-year saved, around 40 times better than the threshold set for health technology assessment by the National Institute for Clinical Excellence.

Non-smoking policies and attitudes to smokers

Individual experience, compounded by knowledge of the apparently low success rates in many short-term studies of smoking cessation, may reinforce a sense of despondency in primary care about trying to help smokers quit the habit, particularly when studies that demonstrate higher rates of sustained quitting have also given a level of support to individuals far beyond that which would be possible in general practice in the UK.

However, stopping smoking does not depend on a single attempt with specific medical assistance or other formal support. More than 90% of successful quitters in the USA do so without any such help. Many smokers make repeated attempts to quit (an average of five or six times) over a long period before success is achieved. One interpretation of these figures is that repeated quit attempts are a learning process and increase the likelihood of eventual long-term success. An alternative and more likely explanation is that they reflect the difficulties that smokers who wish to quit experience in accessing services. The advent of a comprehensive smoking cessation strategy in the UK may help to address problems of service provision, but a more persistent deterrent to access is the widely held perception that attitudes within the health services towards smokers seeking help are too often characterised by frustration and blame.

The quit ratio (i.e. the number of ex-smokers as a percentage of those who have ever regularly smoked) has risen year by year. In the UK it is 47% in men and 44% in women, and has even reached 70% in men over 65 years of age, in whom the rate is admittedly enhanced by loss through mortality suffered by these smokers. Much of this quitting has been achieved without the aid of drugs, which improve rates, although it may be the case that these remaining smokers have higher levels of nicotine dependency and so may be more difficult to help.

The role of primary care in the community can help to create an informative and supportive local environment for potential quitters, while the ability of the primary care team to offer continuity of care places it in a powerful position to support quitters who fail towards eventual success.

The likely bonus is that decreasing the prevalence of smoking in the community will reduce the exposure of others to its passive effects, and will also decrease the likelihood of younger people succumbing to the addiction themselves (*see* Chapter 1).

Attitudes

The overwhelming majority of GPs (96%) and practice nurses (99%) accept that intervening in smoking is part of their role,[3] and most patients (80%) see their GP at least once a year.

Nevertheless, only 29% of smokers who have seen their GP in the previous year recall having been given advice to stop smoking. If this is a true reflection of practice, there may be a number of reasons for it.

- GPs are keen to avoid negative responses from patients and to maintain good relationships.[4] Finding time to address an issue that was not the patient's main reason for coming to see the doctor, in a way that does not threaten the relationship, is difficult.
- The treatment of disease is the dominant focus of most GPs' activity, and their ethos is one of resolving patients' complaints. The confidence of GPs in their own ability to effect a change in smoking behaviour is low.[5,6] Nonetheless, a significant number of consultations will be related to a disease process which, if the person is a smoker, provides a rationale for raising the subject.

GPs' attitudes to prescribing medication to aid smoking cessation are apparently equally discrepant with their acceptance that they have a role in smoking cessation. In a survey published in October 2001, 43% of GPs felt that bupropion should not be available on NHS prescription and 50% felt that nicotine replacement therapy (NRT) should be equally unavailable.[7] In their analysis of the survey, the authors speculated that the reasons for this could include the following:

- failure to accept that nicotine dependence is a genuine medical disorder
- lack of sympathy for a condition that is regarded as self-inflicted
- low absolute efficacy rates for medication.

Previous surveys have suggested that there is a widespread belief that NRT is not cost-effective, despite compelling evidence to the contrary.

In general, the task of helping smokers to quit is somewhat thankless. Lives saved in this way are less visible than those saved by interventions in the more traditional medical territory of acute disease.

Patients themselves are less hesitant about anti-smoking strategies. Most people are in favour of smoking bans at work. A Department of Health study found that the number of people in favour of workplace smoking bans increased from 81% in 1996 to 86% in 2000. A survey in one shopping centre found 88% of respondents in support of a smoking ban. Even smokers were in favour, as 97% were still shopping there and 75% supported the ban.

Policies

The policies and attitudes of the practice set the scene for a smoking cessation service. There is a thin line between stigmatising smokers on the one hand and ignoring them on the other. Achieving a practice culture that is sympathetic to those who want to give up, open and informative for those who do not or cannot, and supportive of those who remain ex- or non-smokers, is a prerequisite for success.

Central to this policy should be the recognition that addiction to nicotine is comparable with addiction to narcotics such as heroin. For most smokers, the first step on this journey to addiction begins as a simple expression of adolescent rebellion, glamour or machismo. The insidious process of addiction is subtly driven by commercial promotion and (although perhaps less so today) by peer group pressure.

Smokers are not to blame for their addiction. Many will need considerable reserves of will-power to quit, whatever support they have.

The primary care team

Premises

The NHS as a whole espouses a non-smoking policy, and there can be few GP premises where smoking remains an option throughout the building. Nevertheless, 28% of the adult patients who come to see their GP are smokers, and if national statistics are at all representative of primary care staff, there are probably also several smokers in each primary healthcare team. As responsible employers, GPs should manage the tension between concerns about passive smoking and the rights of smokers to continue their habit if they wish to do so.

Passive smoking
Exposure to environmental tobacco smoke is a cause of ischaemic heart disease and lung cancer. In the case of the latter, long-term exposure increases the risk by the order of 20–30%.

The task is not made easier by lack of clarity in the legislation. The regulations about non-smoking policies in places of work apply, of course, to practice premises. However, the Health and Safety at Work Act 1974 and EU Directives do not impose a clear duty to ban smoking in the workplace, but only imply a requirement, unless employers can show that it is unreasonable or impractical.

In practice, employment tribunals have generally found in favour of employees who have been forced to leave their jobs on account of exposure to passive smoking. Smokers have also tested their right to smoke, in the courts, but have not been successful.

In the White Paper, 'Smoking Kills', the Government announced its intention to consult on the best methods for tackling the problem.[1] Since that time, an 'Approved Code of Practice' on passive smoking at work has not appeared.

The dual roles of employer and clinician can be difficult to combine, but GPs do have an opportunity to offer cessation support to staff who are both smokers and patients of the practice, and to provide those members of staff who are not registered with the practice with information about smoking cessation services in general. However, staff may need reassurance that their employment status is in no way jeopardised by their smoking status.

In a survey of health at work in primary care by the Health Development Agency in 1998, 91% of practice managers stated that their practice had a smoking policy, and it was found that 51% of these policies were written. In total, 93% of practices banned smoking on the premises, and 72% of practices had written material to help their staff to stop smoking.

A systematic review of the effect of non-smoking policies in public places suggested that those which were likely to have the greatest benefit were 'carefully planned and resourced, multi-component strategies'.

One template for a workplace smoking cessation policy is a draft document from Action on Smoking and Health (ASH), which sets out a framework that may be relatively easily adopted for general practice (see Appendix 5).

Patients

The face that the practice offers to patients is important with regard to overcoming the prejudices of smokers and primary care staff alike. Smokers will seek help if they want to stop (most of them do) and if their perceptions of the practice are that such help is going to be offered non-judgmentally and with enthusiasm. Primary care staff will find it more rewarding to offer a service that is being openly sought, rather than one which is being imposed on an unwilling recipient (with less chance of success). The reality is that enthusiasm about providing the service will diminish if it is grudgingly sought.

There are a number of strategies that can help to develop the practice's 'shop window' in this way.

1 Leaflet and poster advertising can be used in the surgery. Supplies are widely and often freely available (*see* Appendix 6). A useful exercise is to sit in your own waiting area and ask yourself a number of questions. For example, is it clear to smokers:
   - that smoking is harmful to the health of smokers and non-smokers alike?
   - that the practice is a non-smoking area?
   - how they can obtain information about smoking?
   - how they can access help with quitting the habit?
2 Developing links and activities with other organisations with a shared concern about smoking (e.g. schools, local government, self-help groups, patient organisations, and local dentists and chemists).
3 Providing information about other sources of help to smokers (*see* Appendix 6).
4 Promoting a culture of support for smokers within the practice who are trying to quit, in clinical and other meetings.
5 Co-ordinating local/practice publicity with national initiatives. One-third of smokers thought about trying to stop smoking on National No-Smoking Day 2000.

Box 5.1 Raising awareness 1

It became apparent in a practice that many women attending antenatal clinics had never had their smoking status recorded and had never been offered support to stop smoking.

In a simple survey of 26 sets of 'current' antenatal records, less than half had a smoking history recorded in them, and none had a record of being offered support in trying to stop smoking. The midwives in the primary healthcare team (PHCT) organised a meeting with the practice smoking cessation adviser and GPs. It was decided that smoking cessation literature should form part of the package of information that was given to all patients attending first antenatal appointments, and that the subject would be raised in antenatal classes. Particular attention would be paid to raising the topic of smoking cessation during prenatal counselling, and wherever possible referrals for smoking cessation support would be made to the practice smoking cessation adviser. Ensuring that patients' smoking status was known to secondary care in letters of referral and shared records would reinforce the practice's activity. An audit cycle would be developed to monitor progress towards better recording of status and intervention.

Box 5.2 Raising awareness 2

An audit of a smoking cessation clinic in a six-doctor practice of 12 000 patients revealed a disappointingly low attendance rate. Less than three patients per week were attending the nurse-led clinic.

At one of their regular primary healthcare team meetings, a decision was made to provide the smoking cessation lead (a practice nurse) with protected time to identify the reasons for this low attendance and to produce a response. The nurse approached the practice's Patient Participation Group (PPG) and, with their help, developed a brief questionnaire survey for surgery attenders. She also spent time talking to patients, their representatives in the PPG and practice staff individually.

A number of problems were identified, including the following.

- Patients and even some staff in the practice were unaware of the existence of the clinic.
- Patients who had heard of the service were unsure how to gain access to it.
- Staff were also unsure about access issues. The clinic had been set up to provide smokers with open access, but many believed that it was invariably necessary to see a GP first. Many of those patients were anxious about seeking help from their GP, believing that they might receive a negative response.
- The services offered by the clinic were not widely known to would-be users.
- Three members of the staff were smokers, and all of them were keen to stop. The two individuals who were patients of the practice felt ashamed and unable to seek help from the clinic.

A second meeting with the primary healthcare team and the PPG was arranged to present these findings, and a number of strategies were developed.

- Staff who were both smokers and patients of the practice were offered smoking cessation support outside the normal clinic times. By 6 months both were non-smokers.
- The PPG commissioned an article from the smoking cessation lead for its monthly newsletter about the clinic. The newsletter is free, and is available in the surgery and at a number of outlets in the practice area.
- Posters advertising the availability of the clinic were produced, and a campaign began – using these as well as a wide variety of leaflet and poster information about smoking cessation. This information was made available at dental surgeries, schools, and child health and antenatal clinics, as well as at local chemists and the community hospital casualty department. A special effort was made leading up to National No-Smoking Day.
- All members of the primary healthcare team, including health visitors and midwives, were encouraged to promote the availability of the clinic. Referral source data were collected by the clinic and fed back to the team at subsequent meetings.

Three months later it was necessary to make extra clinic time available. Attendance rates have fluctuated since then, but an annual campaign leading up to National No-Smoking Day is now an established part of the practice's calendar.

Reflection exercises

Exercise 9

Visit a neighbouring practice and compare the way in which you tackle helping people to stop smoking in your practice with their systems and procedures. Compare both practices' versions of the 'stop-smoking' protocols while you are there. Discuss any differences or gaps, and refine your protocols accordingly in line with the most recent evidence.

Exercise 10

Review the patient literature you have on diet, smoking, body mass index and weight loss, alcohol consumption and physical activity. How does your literature compare with the up-to-date recommendations for smoking and other evidence-based guidelines for healthy lifestyles?

Ask patients of different ages and backgrounds who smoke, and who are at risk of heart disease or stroke, to look at your patient literature and to let you know whether it is appropriate (i.e. easy to read and relevant) for them. Update your patient educational literature accordingly. Find out what self-help groups might supply more appropriate literature, or download material from suitable websites and photocopy it if it is copyright-free.

Exercise 11

Find out what initiatives have been undertaken by any members of the practice team to ascertain patients' views during the previous 12 months. This might include surveying or involving anyone registered with the practice (regular patients, people who do not use the services, carers) or the local community. How was the information collected from the initiative used? Did changes result?

This exercise will be particularly relevant to the theme of this book if you use the same methodology to investigate the views of people who smoke about the smoking cessation services in your practice. Your own or practice team members' learning needs from this exercise might include the following:

(i) learning more about the range of methods that can be employed to find out patients' views
(ii) learning how to apply any of those methods to ascertain the views of people who smoke, or who have smoking-related conditions, about the care or services that are provided or that they wish to receive
(iii) learning more about the doctor or nurse involving individual patients in decision making about stopping smoking.

Discuss the information that you have obtained with the practice team, and plan how to make improvements in your services.

Now that you have completed these interactive reflection exercises, transfer the information to the relevant section about your learning needs in the empty template on pages 169–178 if you are working on your own personal development plan, or to the practice personal and professional development plan on pages 193–199 if you are working on a practice team learning plan. Don't forget to keep the evidence of your learning in your personal portfolio.

References

1 Department of Health (1998) *Smoking Kills. A White Paper on tobacco.* The Stationery Office, London.

2 Raw M, McNeill A and West R (1998) Smoking cessation guidelines for health professionals: a guide to effective smoking cessation interventions for the healthcare system. *Thorax.* **53** (**Supplement 5**): Part 1, 1–19.

3 McEwen A and West R (2000) Smoking cessation activities by general practitioners and practice nurses. *Tobacco Control.* **10**: 27–32.

4 Coleman T, Murphy E and Cheater F (2000) Factors influencing discussion of smoking between general practitioners and patients who smoke: qualitative study. *Br J Gen Pract.* **50**: 207–10.

5 Steptoe A, Doherty S, Kendrick T, Rink E and Hilton S (1999) Attitudes to cardiovascular health promotion among GPs and practice nurses. *Fam Pract.* **16**: 158–63.

6 McAvoy BR, Kaner EF, Lock CA, Heather N and Gilvarry E (1999) Our Healthier Nation: are general practitioners willing and able to deliver? A survey of attitudes to and involvement in health promotion and lifestyle counselling. *Br J Gen Pract.* **49**: 187–90.

7 McEwen A, West R and Owen L (2001) General practitioners' views on the provision of nicotine replacement therapy and bupropion. *BioMed Central Fam Pract.* **2**: 6.

CHAPTER 6

Opportunities

The overall approach to primary care intervention has been characterised as the xAs, where x varies between 3 and 6 depending on how many steps are described in the process! All approaches have the same intent, namely to establish who is a smoker, to offer information about the risks of smoking , to provide help to those who want to stop and to evaluate the outcome.

Box 6.1 The six As

Ask about smoking at every visit (use a non-directive approach), update the patient's record, and note any interest in stopping.
Advise about the value of stopping and the health risks of continuing to smoke. Use clear appropriate and personalised information. Use open questions (e.g. Have you ever considered stopping? Are you interested in finding out about . . . ?).
Assess willingness to stop (see stages-of-change model).
Assist the patient with planning of the quit attempt. Review past experiences of quit attempts, identify problem areas, enlist support from the patient's family and friends, set a quit date, discuss at-risk moments and lapses, and discuss aids to cessation (e.g. NRT and bupropion).
Arrange follow-up within the practice.
Audit, beginning the audit cycle with simple, achievable standards.

In this chapter we shall discuss the opportunities that arise in primary care to identify and prompt smokers to attempt to stop – Ask, Advise and Assess.

In the next chapter, on interventions, we shall consider the means and mechanisms that can be employed to increase the likelihood of long-term abstinence for both the individual and the practice population – Assist, Arrange and Audit.

Ask

Recording

The 'Gold Standard'
All patients over 16 years of age should have had a record of their
smoking status made within the last year.

A complete record of smoking status may not be obtainable for a variety
of practical reasons.

- At least 80% of patients may attend their practice over the course of
  one year, but 20% do not.
- There is little incentive to re-record non-smoking status annually in
  middle-aged adults who are highly unlikely to take up the habit.
- Registration 'ghosts' still haunt practice registers.
- Many smokers will have started before the age of 16 years, even
  though this is illegal.
- Repeated inquisitions about smoking status are difficult, and they
  can be counter-productive both as a means to smoking cessation and
  in the wider context of primary care.

However, it is impossible to target activity and measure its outcome
without quantifying the problem. Indeed, simply introducing a recording system increases the likelihood of advice being given about stopping
smoking by up to threefold. A record on the computer or in the notes is
an important reminder for future consultations

In one survey,[1] 99% of GPs said that they recorded the smoking
status of all new patients and 57% reported that they regularly updated
patients' records. A study comparing survey results with GP records[2]
found that 74% contained a record of smoking, and the main discrepancy was that 46% were recorded as never having smoked when in fact
they were ex-smokers. Similar data were found in another survey[3] in
which 73% of notes had an entry about smoking made over a 5-year
period. Paradoxically, the main discrepancy was an overestimate of
smoking prevalence. The primary care team is understandably less
interested in history than in status, but ex-smokers are nevertheless
at greater risk of a variety of diseases in the long term, and ignorance of
a patient's current smoking status hinders any consultation in which
better health is the aim.

Patients' own reports of their smoking status may not always be reliable. In one study, 17 out of 260 former smokers with ischaemic heart disease whose smoking status was chemically validated by means of exhaled carbon monoxide measurements and serum cotinine levels were found to be still smoking despite a self-report to the contrary.[4] Unreliable reporting may be more a result of misperception than of deception. Pipe and cigar smokers may not classify themselves as smokers. Even cigarette smokers who have effectively (although usually temporarily) cut down may regard themselves as having stopped the habit. When reviewing the smoking status of high-risk 'ex-smokers' it may be worth making a specific enquiry.

Despite the difficulties of maintaining an accurate register, effective recording of patients' smoking status is an essential precursor to a practice-based smoking cessation programme, and requires a rigorous and methodical approach that is an integral part of the practice's work. Fortunately, computerisation makes this a comparatively easy task.

Read codes

The NHS approved coding system is the hierarchical one of Read codes. There are at least 49 separate Read codes that concern smoking status and associated interventions. Limiting the fields will make it easier both to input the information and, more importantly, to extract relevant and meaningful data subsequently.

When deciding on a strategy for recording it is important to ensure consistency with other clinical activities in the practice that concern smoking cessation.

For example, the National Service Framework for Coronary Heart Disease (NSF CHD) recommends that data about smoking should be a key performance indicator.[5] Collecting data to meet these standards should be approached in a way that is entirely consistent with data entered about smoking in other areas of work. Mapping these overlaps in high-risk groups is a useful first step towards ensuring that protocols in each area have a consistent mechanism for recording smoking status.

The trend towards an agreed national set of Read codes has been driven by the NHS Information Agency. It has been accelerated by innovations such as the software programme MIQUEST, which has been endorsed by the NHS Executive as the recommended method for expressing queries and extracting data from different types of practice systems using a common set of Read codes. Local audit groups and primary care organisations are useful reference sources when developing a practice system.

What should be recorded?

Decide on a small number of codes with which the whole primary healthcare team can become familiar. One way of ensuring consistency of recording is to set up templates or create common entries specific to the practice.

There are two versions of Read codes, namely 4 byte and version 2 (which has up to five alphanumerical characters), as well as a range of practice electronic record systems, including those from computer systems EMIS, TOREX and VAMP, but the basic principle of keeping data entry focused on clearly defined outcomes at the outset remains the same.

The codes listed in Tables 6.1 and 6.2 are those used in our own practice, and are variously recommended by the local medical audit

Table 6.1 Read codes for smoking status

If possible (e.g. on EMIS systems), record code plus number of cigarettes per day	137 . . . plus value
Current smoker	137R
Never smoked	1371
Current non-smoker	137L
Trivial smoker (< 1 cigarette per day)	1372
Light smoker (1–9 cigarettes per day)	1373
Moderate smoker (10–19 cigarettes per day)	1374
Heavy smoker (20–39 cigarettes per day)	1375
Very heavy smoker (> 40 cigarettes per day)	1376
Pipe smoker	137H

Table 6.2 Read codes for smoking cessation interventions

Health education on smoking (*for any advice given by a primary healthcare team member*)	6791
Stop-smoking monitoring (*for any in-practice referral for stopping smoking, i.e. to practice smoking cessation adviser*)	9OO (capital letter O)
Attends stop-smoking monitoring (*any referral to specialist smoking cessation clinic outside primary healthcare team*)	9OO1
Refuses stop-smoking monitoring (*for any refusal to be referred or did not attend in or outside the practice*)	9OO2

advisory group, primary care organisation and smoking cessation services.

For non-cigarette smokers the amount smoked can be recorded in 'cigarette equivalents' (*see* Box 6.2). Although this is a less than satisfactory way of ascertaining the total daily consumption of nicotine (which may, for example, vary widely between different sizes of 'large' cigar), it has the virtue of simplifying data entry. The practice may want to revisit this issue when the routine of recording smoking status is established.

Box 6.2 Cigarette equivalents

Pipe smokers
One bowl = 2.5 cigarettes

Cigars
One small cigar = 1.5 cigarettes
One medium-sized cigar = 2 cigarettes
One large cigar = 4 cigarettes

'Roll-ups'
1 oz (25 g) tobacco = 50 cigarettes

Who will record it and when?

Almost all members of the primary healthcare team can be involved in entering smoking cessation data, and the opportunities to do so are so ubiquitous that there is a risk of becoming swamped by the attempt.

First steps might include the following.

- Raise the profile of data entry with the whole team whenever the opportunity presents itself.
- Make the recommended codes widely available in hard-copy and electronic versions.
- Incorporate the recommended codes into existing computer and written protocols.
- Initially concentrate on areas where current smoking poses a particularly high risk to the patient (e.g. cardiovascular disease, diabetes, pregnancy).

Box 6.3 The Smoking Cherub

The primary healthcare team was becoming increasingly frustrated by their apparent inability to achieve their audit standards for recording smoking status data. When reasons such as lack of time, wrong Read codes and other data collection problems had all been exhausted, it was still found that data entry was incomplete. The issue was distilled into one of motivation, and the solution was one of 'carrot or stick'.

The practice manager purchased a small trophy (an idiosyncratic choice of a glass ball surrounded by gold-coloured plastic cherubs!). The day before each primary healthcare team meeting, smoking status data entry figures for each member of the team were produced. At the meeting the award was made to the member of the team with the highest proportion of key data entries to patients seen. Competition for 'The Smoking Cherub' increased data entry by 50% between the first and second meetings! (Post-modern ironic sensibility or the inherent desire to win?)

Advise

Around 80% of patients will consult their GP in any one year, and approximately 1–2% of patients who smoke will quit and remain abstinent after 6 months if simply advised to do so by their doctors.[6] If GPs were to advise a further 50% of smokers to stop, and to provide them with NRT or Zyban, according to existing protocols, there could be an additional 75 000 ex-smokers in the UK each year. In other words, a relatively small investment of time could yield a considerable and worthwhile return.

Extrapolations such as this provide an apparently compelling reason for not only asking all patients at every opportunity about their smoking status, *but also advising them to stop.*

However, many GPs feel uncomfortable with this blunt approach. Only 30% of GPs in one survey[7] thought it practicable to advise smokers to stop on every occasion. Despite the understandable gaps between giving advice, hearing it and remembering it, if smokers' recollections are even an approximation to actual practice, GPs are not always 'asking and advising'. There may be benefits in discriminating between smokers who are likely to be receptive to advice and those who are not. Some evidence suggests that giving advice to those who are not ready to change may be unhelpful and entrench unhealthy behaviour.

It has been estimated that 20% of existing smokers are ready to quit, 40% are unsure and 40% are not ready to quit. Smokers claim that there is a fulcrum between 'readiness' to quit and willingness to 'go for it'. Although this equilibrium is shifting and ill defined, advice and support given at this point is perhaps most likely to tip the balance towards a serious quitting attempt. Behaviour change at any time is not easy, and smokers are no exception to this.

In one qualitative study,[8] patients were often found to have made their own evaluations about smoking, and they did not believe that doctors' advice could influence them. They felt that quitting was 'down to them'. They anticipated that doctors would offer advice, and they could respond as 'contrary', 'matter of fact' or 'self-blaming'. The study concluded that doctors should tailor their approach to the patient, and that interventions should be sympathetic and not repeated or ritualistic (which may be counterproductive).

Box 6.4 Cutting down

GPs' awareness of the factors that could entrench smoking behaviour or increase resistance to advice to stop may underlie the perpetuation of advice to 'cut down' as a way round the starker issue of stopping altogether.

Reducing the amount smoked is unlikely to be useful. Smokers compensate by smoking more intensively, and almost invariably resume their normal consumption eventually. As a strategy it risks alleviating the pressure to stop entirely. For this reason, the available guidelines focus entirely on total quitting.

An unthinking 'blanket' approach to intervention may be counterproductive. Smoking cessation interventions may be most effective when they are focused on those who are ready to change and those at high risk – recognising that the latter often include the former! Advice seems to be best aimed not so much at persuading smokers to stop as at triggering an attempt to quit.[9]

Inviting smokers to make the attempt and then waiting for a response (e.g. a later telephone request for support) may be a sensible sifting approach for determining who is motivated.

Assess

In a paper published in 1983, Prochaska and DiClemente[10] proposed the *stages-of-change* model (*see* Box 6.5) as best representing smokers' readiness to quit. Theoretically the model has its faults. However, a measure of its utility is that it has been almost universally incorporated into most smoking cessation strategies. Of particular relevance to primary care is the fact that, rather than using limited time and resources to cajole a reluctant patient into a best-fit quitting plan, the emphasis is on identifying the patient who is ready to quit, and then working with them rather than against them.

Box 6.5 The stages-of-change model

1 *Pre-contemplation*: Patients do not recognise that they have a problem, and are likely to resist or avoid a confrontational approach. A better strategy is to 'agree to disagree', offer educational advice in a non-pejorative way, and suggest that you reassess their attitude to stopping smoking at some point in the future (i.e. remember that people change!).

2 *Contemplation*: The contemplator recognises that they have a problem, but equivocates over a commitment to quit. Pushing against their ambivalence is unlikely to succeed. Acknowledge their uncertainties and reassure them that this is a recognised part of the process of becoming a non-smoker. Offer information that will help the patient to reason for him- or herself (e.g. help them to assemble a list of 'pros and cons' of smoking).

3 *Action*: The patient is ready and keen to make a quit attempt. Develop a plan.

4 *Maintenance*: Around 70% of patients who quit relapse within 3 months, but this figure can improve with support, perhaps through follow-up telephone calls, advanced warning about withdrawal, adjusting pharmacotherapy as appropriate, or developing strategies in advance for dealing with at-risk times.

5 *Relapse*: Reassure don't censure. Help the patient to regard it as an opportunity from which they can learn. Offer to support them in another attempt. Most smokers try several times before quitting for good.

The practical, primary care skills of screening, brief intervention and patient-centred planning of care dovetail neatly into this model, and can provide a clinically effective and efficient use of consultation time.

GPs do not accept that they should give advice to stop smoking at every opportunity and there is evidence that repeatedly giving advice to the same smoker reduces the likelihood of their stopping.[11] In general, GPs show a preference for offering advice to smokers with smoking-related disease[9] and, even though they do not respond better than others,[11] smokers are more receptive to advice when it is linked to a medical condition, whether or not the latter is smoking-related.[8] In this context, GPs may also feel more confident about using a more overtly 'problem-solving' approach. Eliciting patients' beliefs about the effects of smoking on their health may be a useful indirect measure of their willingness to make a quitting attempt. When smokers attribute their respiratory symptoms to smoking, they are six times more likely to intend to stop smoking.[12]

Box 6.6 The teachable moment

It comes when least expected. It is not planned, but it should always be anticipated – that wonderful, serendipitous teachable moment, when student and teacher come together and it's *carpe diem*!

Jean Ramirez, Language Academy Field Supervisor

Assessing a patient's medical, social and emotional situation in order to provide timely, effective and appropriate intervention is a particular skill and signal responsibility of GPs. Not infrequently there is a brief window of opportunity for the professional that coincides with receptivity in the patient. The ability to identify and capitalise on these 'teachable moments' hinges on the unique ability of primary care to offer continuity of care combined with knowledge of the patients' past medical, family and social history.

Such 'moments' may be as obvious as part of a patient's rehabilitation after myocardial infarction, or as subtle as the knowledge that the uncle of a young smoker has recently been diagnosed with lung cancer, or that the father of a wheezy baby is a smoker. It may even extend to suggesting that they influence a family member's behaviour.

Teachable moments may be too many and too elusive to itemise, but more can be said about the contexts within which they are likely to occur, which include the following:

1 smoking-related illness (e.g. chronic obstructive airways disease)
2 the 'worried well' smoker (e.g. in pregnancy, prenatal counselling)
3 anticipatory care (e.g. passive smoking).

Smoking-related illness

For a more detailed account of the association between disease and smoking, *see* Chapter 2. In this section some examples of smoking-related disease will be discussed inasmuch as they present an opportunity for the health professional to offer support with a quitting attempt. Two opportunities arise when smoking cessation advice may be more than usually effective – at or around the point of diagnosis and during the period of chronic disease monitoring. The organisation of much of this activity into clinics that run to a practice protocol usefully focuses smoking cessation interventions on those who are most at risk.

Cardiovascular disease

Smoking contributes to 30% of all ischaemic heart disease deaths, and doubles the risk of stroke. Stopping smoking reduces the risk of subsequent events.

Not only do cardiac events and procedures encourage smokers to quit,[13] but preoperative interventions and post-discharge follow-up do so as well. Cessation rates at 1 year in patients who have been hospitalised with a coronary condition are around 50%,[14] and the worse the symptoms of disease, the more likely patients are to quit.[15,16] Patients with an initial infarct who stop smoking have a 50% lower risk of reinfarction, sudden cardiac death and total mortality.[17] Transdermal NRT patches are safe for patients with ischaemic heart disease.[18] However, there are warnings on most forms of NRT about their use in such patients, and it may still be wise to obtain informed consent from the patient before a quitting attempt is made under medical supervision.

In their submission in September 2001 to the expected National Institute for Clinical Excellence appraisal of smoking cessation drugs, Action on Smoking and Health (ASH) stated:

> There are very considerable gains in reducing risk of heart disease and stroke through smoking cessation – even if nicotine itself increases these risks. We support recommendations from the new guidelines in press that NRT can normally be recommended to smokers with CVD who tried and failed

to quit without such help. In all cases of CVD – no matter how severe – there is a case for offering NRT in the situation where the patient is continuing to smoke. In severe cases, the warnings imply that it would be dangerous, but this can never be more dangerous and will always be considerably less dangerous than continued smoking. We recommend that in severe CVD cases the specialist is advised to make a risk–benefit judgement that takes full account of the mortal risk of continued smoking when deciding what drugs to offer to assist smoking cessation.

There is also evidence that bupropion is safe to use in patients with cardiovascular disease and improves abstinence rates over six months.[19]

Not only does proven ischaemic heart disease encourage patients to make a quitting attempt and improve quit rates, but also a study found that 75% of patients with chest pain of whatever origin in a US emergency room[20] indicated their willingness to take part in smoking cessation interventions. The attitudes of patients in the UK are currently being researched, but it seems unlikely that they will be significantly different.

Chronic obstructive airways disease

Chronic obstructive airways disease is largely preventable and is primarily linked to smoking. The lifetime risk of the disease is low in non-smokers (5% in one large study[21]). The airflow obstruction in chronic obstructive pulmonary disease is usually progressive in individuals who continue to smoke. This results in early disability and shortened survival times.

If the impairment of forced expiratory volume (FEV_1) is moderate, stopping smoking can revert the decline in lung function to the values found in non-smokers,[22] and there is a reduction in cough, phlegm and wheeze. Most benefits seem to occur during the first year. If lung function is more severely impaired, the effects of smoking cessation are less certain, and to obtain reductions in morbidity and mortality due to chronic obstructive pulmonary disease, stopping smoking early is necessary.

NRT is safe in patients with chronic obstructive pulmonary disease (COPD), and bupropion SR is also an effective aid to smoking cessation in individuals with mild to moderate COPD.[23]

Diabetes

The prevalence of smoking amongst people with diabetes (types I and II) seems to differ little from that in the general population (around 25%). Sadly, the fact that smoking prevalence decreases with the duration of the disease is probably related to premature death rather than to success in stopping smoking.

Smoking and diabetes are both independently strong risk factors for macrovascular disease, and several studies have shown that impairment of renal function, the development of neuropathy and possibly retinopathy are all adversely associated with smoking.

In one study of cost-effectiveness,[24] counselling smokers to stop was found to be more cost-effective than treating hypertension or screening for high cholesterol levels. The implication, as yet unsupported by evidence, is that smoking cessation activities in diabetic patients are likely to be all the more cost-effective.

In many smokers, fears about weight gain are referred to as reasons for not quitting, and there is evidence to suggest that diabetics regard smoking as a strategy for controlling both their weight and their diabetes.[25] Providing information about the relative risks of weight gain and smoking is of particular value in the setting of a diabetic clinic.

NRT is not contraindicated in otherwise uncomplicated diabetes. However, in patients with diabetes that is being treated with hypoglycaemic agents, which potentially lower the seizure threshold, Medicines Control Agency guidelines advise that bupropion should only be prescribed if clinical circumstances are compelling.

Cancer

Most GPs will see relatively few newly diagnosed patients with cancer each year, and those whom they do see will of course have different prognoses, but in general patients who are being treated for cancer are now surviving longer.

Clearly the diagnosis of a smoking-related cancer is a strong incentive for patients to attempt to quit, and at some if not several points in the cancer journey there are likely to be 'teachable moments'. However, even in these circumstances, over one-third of patients continue to smoke after the attempt. For some the association between smoking and cancer may be unclear (e.g. pancreatic, bladder and cervical cancers). In others, having developed cancer, the patient may feel that the benefits of stopping no longer apply. In the latter group there is accumulating evidence that stopping reduces the risks of recurrence, second cancers and the development of pre-malignant conditions,[26] and that it improves survival rates.[27]

Worried well smokers

Pregnancy

Asking about smoking status should be a routine part of prenatal care (asking about smoking and the pill) and antenatal counselling and screening. Smoking status should be highlighted on antenatal records and advice offered about the risks of continued smoking, together with support for quit attempts, including referral to the specialist smoking cessation service. Group sessions during pregnancy have been reported to be very poorly attended in most trials, and are probably not justified.[28] Although relapse prevention seems to be relatively ineffective during the postnatal period, advice that this is a high-risk time, together with the offer of further support, may be of benefit.

Circumstances in and around the time of pregnancy present particular challenges and opportunities with regard to smoking cessation interventions.

1 Prenatally there is evidence that smoking increases the time to conception.[29] During pregnancy, women are highly motivated because of concern about their babies and they are in regular contact with the healthcare system. They are likely to obtain higher levels of social and family support for attempting to stop smoking at this time, and they may be all the more motivated if a partner who smokes is willing to make a quitting attempt as well.
BUT
Health care providers of routine care generally perform poorly in antenatal interventions to stop women smoking, although midwives deliver interventions at a higher rate than doctors. There is a strong social gradient, with continuing smokers tending to be socially disadvantaged.
2 Up to 25% of women who smoke before pregnancy have stopped by the time they have their first antenatal appointment.
BUT
'Victim blaming' may lead to under-reporting of smoking in

pregnancy, and 25% of mothers will have started smoking again during pregnancy.
3 Quitting early in pregnancy or prenatally gives the most health benefits.
BUT
Quitting at any time during or before pregnancy is of benefit.

Of those who are still smoking at the time of the first antenatal appointment, about 10% will stop with usual care and a further 6–7% will stop with a smoking cessation programme. Overall, interventions to help pregnant women quit smoking produce an absolute difference of 8.1% in validated late-pregnancy quit rates.[30]

If complete abstinence cannot be achieved, it is likely that a 50% reduction in smoking would be the minimum necessary to benefit the health of mother and baby. Relapse prevention programmes have shown little success during the postpartum period. This is a situation in which the more generally applied maxim that cutting down is probably of no benefit may not apply. In this instance it is the baby who clearly benefits, rather than the pregnant smoker.

Again there are inconsistencies in product labelling and advice. Some forms of NRT are contraindicated in pregnant women, while others can be used on medical advice, or following a medical assessment of the risk–benefit ratio, if the pregnant woman has tried and failed to give up smoking without nicotine substitution.

Expert opinion is that despite the risks of nicotine in pregnancy, NRT is considerably safer than continued smoking in pregnancy,[31] which also exposes the fetus and mother to many other toxins in addition to nicotine.

Nicotine replacement therapy is effective in pregnancy. There is a confusing range of (probably flawed) advice, but it should:

- only be made available to the heaviest smokers
- only be considered in women who smoke more than 10 cigarettes a day and who have made a recent unsuccessful attempt to quit without replacement therapy.

Relevant guidance can be summarised as follows.

- Requiring a pregnant smoker to try stopping without NRT first is unhelpful. Failure risks demotivating the patient, who may then continue to smoke throughout the pregnancy.
- The contraindication to NRT in pregnancy will hopefully be removed and pregnant smokers advised to use NRT if their prospects of quitting without it are poor.

- Theoretically, a 16-hour NRT patch is safer for the fetus than a 24-hour patch, as nicotine levels should be lower than when the patient is smoking, although in neither case are the additional toxins provided by cigarettes present.
- Bupropion is not currently recommended in pregnancy.

The pill and smoking

Reports of a link between combined oral contraceptive (COC) use and myocardial infarction appeared soon after the pill was first marketed in the 1960s. By the late 1970s, epidemiological studies had confirmed the risk, particularly in smokers using 50 mcg oestrogen preparations. The relative risk estimate for COC users was between 2- to 5-fold greater than in non-users, and 20- to 30-fold greater for COC users who smoked heavily compared with women who did not use COCs and were non-smokers.

Over the years, manufacturers have progressively lowered the doses, developed new progestins and devised new formulations, such as triphasic preparations that release different doses of oestrogen and progestin over the course of the menstrual cycle. Use of current COCs has little or no influence on the risk of a non-fatal first myocardial infarction among women who do not smoke or who smoke less than 25 cigarettes a day. However, concurrent COC use together with heavy smoking increases the risk of myocardial infarction to a level about 30 times that for non-smokers who do not use COCs.

New or repeat attendances related to COC prescribing provide a useful opportunity to update records about smoking status and offer educational advice and smoking cessation support. In older women who are heavy smokers and who are unable or unwilling to stop, and where there may be other risk factors for myocardial ischaemia, alternative methods of contraception may be appropriate.

Although it may be difficult to raise the subject, appointments at which contraception is discussed also offer an opportunity to talk about the risks of smoking to future fertility.

Anticipatory care

Passive smoking

In children, passive smoking has been linked to sudden infant death syndrome, respiratory tract infection, middle ear effusion and decreased lung function. Regulating to reduce their exposure to smoking in schools and public places in this context is unhelpful. Children in smokers' households are not only exposed to risk passively, but tend to model themselves on their parents and are more likely to become smokers themselves. Increasing smoking cessation in adults may reduce smoking uptake in children.

Any proposal to legislate against smoking at home is highly unlikely to get on to the statute book. Reducing most of the passive exposure to smoke depends on educational and behavioural measures.

The presentation of children with, for example, asthma, recurrent ear infections, glue ear or frequent upper respiratory tract infections provides an opportunity to update the smoking status record of the parents and to offer educational advice, with smoking cessation support where appropriate. For those who are unable or unwilling to stop, the provision of a separate ventilated room might be suggested as one way of reducing their children's risk.

Smokers children tend to become smokers themselves. Efforts to reduce the risk of passive inhalation and later addiction are a worthwhile, if long-term strategy. However, only in the second half of this century will attempts to stop smoking in young people manifestly affect mortality rates.

Patients in secondary care

Among the exceptions to smoking-related illness and the worried well smoker are patients in secondary care, most of whom will have been referred by their GPs.

Earlier mention was made of evidence to suggest that illness, or the possibility of illness (whatever its cause), may increase the receptivity of patients to advice to stop smoking. Referral to hospital, whether acute or chronic, will hopefully provoke the reflex to record smoking status, although some surveys have shown that information about this, is often lacking in referral letters.

 Brief behavioural interventions by hospital staff aimed at inpatient smokers have been disappointing in cardiac[31] and antenatal patients.[32] However, the opportunity remains for primary care teams and the specialist smoking cessation services to capitalise on teachable moments that may arise from these patients' experiences. Busy hospital staff without specialist smoking cessation skills are at a disadvantage. The evidence that supports behavioural interventions and counselling as a means of achieving long-term success stems from studies which show that this support needs to be extensive and delivered by trained staff.[33] However, a systematic review[34] has shown that intensive intervention (inpatient contact plus follow-up for at least 1 month) was associated with a significantly higher cessation rate compared with controls. The development of joint programmes, which are initiated in secondary care and followed up in primary care, is likely to be the most successful strategy for hospitalised smokers. In a primary care setting there is a greater opportunity to offer advice based on models such as that of the stages of change, which can trigger a quit attempt, rather than the necessarily untargeted approach that is adopted in a hospital ward. Follow-up by specialist and intermediate trained smoking cessation advisers with appropriate pharmacotherapy can then best support patients and offer a greater likelihood of successful continued abstinence.

Reflection exercise

Exercise 12

Undertake a SWOT (strengths, weaknesses, opportunities and threats) analysis of the way in which your practice identifies smokers and prompts them to attempt to stop. Alternatively, focus down and look at how the practice operates its systems and procedures for managing patients who smoke who have established smoking-related conditions. This will involve convening a group to represent all elements of your practice team (e.g. GP, nurse, manager/support staff, pharmacist). Then brainstorm what your strengths, weaknesses, opportunities and threats are with respect to the care of such smokers. You will be considering the following:

(i) your infrastructure – the practice protocol, access to and availability of nurse-led clinics, hardware and software, information resources and the capacity for computerised recall

(ii) your capability – staff numbers and posts, skills (e.g. clinical, personal, communication, IT)

(iii) your capacity – how you cope with demand (e.g. if the nurses run the smoking cessation services, who does the work that they did before?)

(iv) the extent to which you work as a team across the practice, with others from secondary care or the independent sector, and most of all with patients, including responding to feedback in order to achieve patient-centred care.

You could use the 14 components of clinical governance described in Chapter 8 as a checklist for the SWOT analysis.

Then make a plan for improvement, including what you need to learn, what you need to buy, who you need to appoint or involve and what you need to reorganise.

Now that you have completed this interactive reflection exercise, transfer the information to the empty template of the personal development plan on pages 169–178 if you are working on your own learning plan, or to the practice personal and professional development plan on pages 193–199 if you are working on a practice team learning plan. Don't forget to keep the evidence of your learning in your personal portfolio.

References

1 McEwen A and West R (2000) Smoking cessation activities by general practitioners and practice nurses. *Tobacco Control.* **10**: 27–32.
2 Mant J, Murphy M, Rose P and Vessey M (2000) The accuracy of general practitioner records of smoking and alcohol use: comparison with patient questionnaires. *J Publ Health Med.* **22**(2): 198–201.
3 Wilson A, Manku-Scott T, Shepherd D and Jones B (2000) A comparison of individual and population smoking data from a postal survey and general practice records. *Br J Gen Pract.* **50**: 465–8.
4 Attebring M, Herlitz J, Berndt A-K *et al.* (2001) Are patients truthful about their smoking habits? A validation of self-report about smoking cessation with biochemical markers of smoking activity amongst patients with ischaemic heart disease. *J Intern Med.* **249**: 145–51.
5 Department of Health (2000) *National Service Framework for Coronary Heart Disease.* The Stationery Office, London.
6 Silagy C and Ketteridge S (1996) The effectiveness of physician advice to aid smoking cessation. In: T Lancaster and C Silagy (eds) *Tobacco Module of the Cochrane Database of Sytematic Reviews. The Cochrane Collaboration: Issue 3.* Update Software, Oxford.
7 McEwen A, Akotia N and West R (2001) General practitioners' views on the English national smoking cessation guidelines. *Addiction.* **96**: 997–1000.
8 Butler CC, Pill R and Stott N (1998) Qualitative study of patients' perceptions of doctors' advice to quit smoking: implications for opportunistic health promotion. *BMJ.* **316**: 1878–81.

9 Coleman T and Wilkinson A (1999) Factors associated with the provision of anti-smoking advice by general practitioners. *Br J Gen Pract.* **49**: 557–8.

10 Prochaska JO and DiClemente CC (1983) Stages and processes of self-change of smoking: toward an integrative model of change. *J Consult Clin Psychol.* **51**: 390–5.

11 Senore C, Battista RN, Shapiro SH *et al.* (1998) Predictors of smoking cessation following physicians' counselling. *Prev Med.* **27**: 412–21.

12 Walters N and Coleman T (2002) Comparisons of the smoking behaviour and attitude of smokers who attribute respiratory symptoms to smoking with those who do not. *Br J Gen Pract.* **52**: 132–4.

13 DeBusk RF, Miller NH, Superko HR *et al.* (1994) A case management system for coronary risk factor modification after acute myocardial infarction. *Ann Intern Med.* **120**: 721–9.

14 Ockene IS, Miller NH and Houston N (1997) Cigarette smoking, cardio-vascular disease and stroke: a statement for health care professionals from the American Heart Association. *Circulation.* **96**: 3243–7.

15 Frid D, Ockene IS, Ockene JK *et al.* (1991) Severity of angiographically proven coronary artery disease predicts smoking cessation. *Am J Prev Med.* **7**: 131–5.

16 Wilhelmsson C, Vedin JA, Elmfeldt D *et al.* (1975) Smoking and myocardial infarction. *Lancet.* **i**: 415–20.

17 Salonen JT (1980) Stopping smoking and long-term mortality after acute myocardial infarction. *Br Heart J.* **43**: 463–9.

18 Working Group for the Study of Transdermal Nicotine in Patients with Coronary Artery Disease (1994) Nicotine replacement therapy for patients with coronary artery disease. *Arch Intern Med.* **154**: 989–95.

19 Tonstad S, Murphy M and Townsend J, on behalf of the Zyban Cardio-vascular Study Team (2001) *Effectiveness and tolerability of Zyban in smokers with cardiovascular disease: week 52 follow-up phase results.* Presented at European Society for Cardiology, 2 September 2001.

20 Bock BC, Becker B, Niaura R and Partridge R (2000) Smoking among emergency chest pain patients: motivation to quit, risk perception and physician intervention. *Nicotine Tobacco Res.* **2**: 93–6.

21 American Thoracic Society (1995) Standards for the diagnosis and care of patients with chronic obstructive pulmonary disease: ATS statement. *Am J Resp Crit Care Med.* **152**: S77–120.

22 Anthonisen NR, Connett JE, Kiley JP *et al.* (1994) Effects of smoking intervention and the use of an inhaled anticholinergic bronchodilator on the rate of decline of FEV_1: the Lung Health Study. *JAMA.* **272**: 1497–505.

23 Tashkin D, Kanner R, Bailey W *et al.* (2001) Smoking cessation in patients with chronic obstructive pulmonary disease: a double-blind, placebo-controlled trial. *Lancet.* **357**: 1571–5.

24 Cummings S, Rubin S and Oster G (1989) The cost-effectiveness of counselling smokers to quit. *JAMA.* **261**: 75–9.

25 Haire-Joshu D, Heady S, Thomas L, Schechtman K and Fisher EB Jr

(1994) Beliefs about smoking and diabetes care. *Diabetes Educ.* **20**: 410–15.

26 US Department of Health and Human Services (1990) *The Health Benefits of Smoking Cessation: a Report of the Surgeon General.* US DHHS Publication No (CDC) 90-8416. US Department of Health and Human Services, Rockville, MD.

27 Gritz ER, Carr CR, Rapkin D *et al.* (1993) Predictors of long-term smoking cessation in head and neck cancer patients. *Cancer Epidemiol Biomarkers Prev.* **2**: 261–70.

28 Lumley J, Oliver S and Waters E (2001) Interventions for promoting smoking cessation during pregnancy (Cochrane Review). In: *The Cochrane Library, Issue 4.* Update Software, Oxford.

29 Munafo M, Murphy M, Whiteman D and Hey K (2002) Does cigarette smoking increase time to conception? *J Biosoc Sci.* **34**: 65–73.

30 Benowitz N (1991) Nicotine replacement therapy during pregnancy. *JAMA* **22**: 3174–7.

31 Hajek P, Taylor PZ and Mills P (2002) Brief intervention during hospital admission to help patients give up after myocardial infarction and bypass surgery: randomised controlled trial. *BMJ.* **324**: 87–9.

32 Hajek P, West R, Lee A *et al.* (2001) Randomised controlled trial of a midwife-delivered brief smoking cessation intervention in pregnancy. *Addiction.* **96**: 485–94.

33 West R (2002) Helping patients in hospital to quit smoking. *BMJ.* **324**: 64.

34 Munafo M, Rigotti N, Lancaster T, Stead L and Murphy M (2001) Interventions for smoking cessation in hospitalised patients: a systematic review. *Thorax.* **56**: 656–63.

CHAPTER 7

Interventions

This chapter continues the theme of the 'six As' (*see* Chapter 6), and is a discussion of three further issues concerning the management of the patient who wishes to stop smoking, and the practice organisation that facilitates this. These are characterised as Assist, Arrange and Audit.

Assist

A planned smoking cessation attempt is less likely to fail than an impulsive one. Helping patients to work through a personal plan not only increases their likelihood of success, but reinforces their motivation and (despite the apparent length of the following list of suggestions) need not be a time-consuming process. Much of the 'work' can be undertaken by the patient prior to an appointment when the plan is summarised with the help of the practice smoking cessation adviser (see below). A systematic approach to this should include a review of the following:

- the patient's smoking diary – look for important cigarettes (e.g. the first cigarette of the day, social links with smoking 'in the pub', after a meal, and at times of stress)
- previous quit attempts – identify particular difficulties experienced in the past (e.g. weight gain, irritability, restlessness, insomnia)
- other at-risk situations (e.g. associations with family and friends who smoke)

Strategies for dealing with at-risk times include the following:

- considering alternatives (e.g. keeping low-calorie snacks in the fridge)
- other lifestyle changes (e.g. taking up a gentle substitute exercise regime – a walk round the block after one's evening meal is a disincentive to smoking)

- listing the patient's reasons for stopping so that they can refer to it at times of temptation
- incentives and rewards (e.g. reserving the money that they would have spent on cigarettes for a personal treat)
- enlisting the support of non-smoking family and/or friends and, if possible, recruiting other family members who smoke to make a joint quit attempt.

Other tasks, including the setting of a quit date, are considered below.

Arrange

The UK has been well ahead of many other countries in providing a national network of services to help smokers to quit. In total, £10 million were made available for the development of services in England in 1999–2000, and £20 million the following year. A total of £30 million is planned for 2002–3.

Box 7.1 NHS smoking cessation services

Measures of cost-effectiveness are compelling. Between April 2000 and March 2001, 126 800 smokers made a quit attempt with the support of the NHS specialist smoking cessation service. According to one estimate of cost-effectiveness,[1] this was at a cost of £209 per patient. Approximately 11% of these will have become lifelong quitters. The cost per life-year saved is less than £800. In comparison, the anti-obesity drug Orlistat was estimated by the National Institute for Clinical Excellence (NICE) to save quality-adjusted life-years at a cost of £46 000. The NICE benchmark cost-effectiveness figure is thought to be around £30 000. Smoking cessation services are 40–50 times better than this.

Such estimates and comparisons may be tedious but they are also crucial. The simpler things may be hard to achieve, but are of almost inestimable value!

An important part of this service development has been training for primary care (*see* Chapter 6), in particular to develop the role of a smoking cessation adviser (SCA) in each team.

The responsibilities of the SCA include the following:

- developing a system for recording smoking status which can be used by the whole primary healthcare team
- developing and maintaining practice protocols
- offering support to members of the team and helping them to meet their training needs
- taking referrals for smoking cessation interventions from the primary care team
- maintaining links with, for example, network meetings of other SCAs and smoking cessation strategies in areas outside primary care.

The advantages of offering the service in a clinic setting have been illustrated in a range of other practice activities. The SCA will require protected time to develop and monitor the service, as well as for training updates and maintaining links with the specialist service.

The specialist service has three tiers. The organisation of smoking cessation activities in the practice should be based on a written protocol that makes appropriate use of these three levels (*see* Appendix 4).

The primary healthcare team

For smokers of less than 10 cigarettes a day, or those who are reluctant to engage with either more intensive support or medication, it may be sufficient to undertake their quit attempt solely with the involvement of an appropriate member of the primary healthcare team, whether they be a GP, practice nurse or midwife. Before attempting this, some assessment of the likelihood of success should be made based on the patient's motivation and level of addiction. Brief opportunistic advice with written information and contact details for other sources of support should precede the setting of a target quit date. Arrangements for follow-up by appointment or by telephone should be made soon after the quit date, and ideally 3 months later as well, with arrangements to record the long-term outcome at 1 year.

Box 7.2 Key elements of a practice protocol

All members should:

- record smoking status, interventions and outcome
- offer brief advice opportunistically
- encourage the appropriate use of NRT or, if this has been unsuccessful in the past, Zyban

---

> - refer patients to the practice smoking cessation adviser for intermediate support
> - publicise the availability of smoking cessation support within and outside the practice
> - make available printed information on smoking cessation.

The smoking cessation adviser (SCA)

Motivated smokers should be able to access this service directly or by referral from other members of the team. SCAs are asked to keep records of all of their interventions and outcomes.

Box 7.3 Key elements of the smoking cessation adviser's work

- Appointments with the SCA of duration 10–30 minutes.
- Explaining and administering prescribed NRT and bupropion.
- Arranging follow-up 4 weeks after the quit date.
- Completing and returning monitoring forms to the smoking advice service.
- Referring smokers to the smoking advice service when appropriate.

The particular advantages of a practice clinic setting for chronic disease monitoring are well documented, and they apply equally well to smoking cessation activity. The model set out here is not intended to be prescriptive, but it does have the advantage of being tried and tested.

Patients who contact the practice for smoking cessation support are asked to keep a diary of their smoking patterns, including the time of day when each cigarette was smoked, why it was smoked, and what else they might have done instead.

An initial 20-minute appointment of 20 minutes with the smoking cessation adviser should cover the following areas:

- smoking history – including the amount smoked, previous quit attempts, and evaluating with the patient the risks vs. benefits of quitting
- review of the current smoking pattern with the diary, considering alternative activities to smoking
- other risk factors for smoking-related disease

- obtaining a baseline measure of exhaled carbon monoxide (*see* Appendix 2)
- discussion of NRT and bupropion, including completion of check-lists for relative and absolute contraindications. Only trained nurse prescribers should issue NRT, otherwise prescriptions are issued by GPs and the ultimate responsibility for providing a prescription rests with them
- setting a target quit date, usually about 1 week later, and giving advice on preparing for it
- providing NRT for 2 weeks or bupropion for 1 month
- advising about other sources of support (e.g. Quitline) (*see* Appendix 6).

A 1-week follow-up appointment (for 10 minutes) should cover the following:

- carbon monoxide measurement
- discussion of slips/lapses
- motivational support
- recording the quit attempt
- issuing 2 weeks' supply of NRT.

A 1-month appointment (for 10 minutes) should cover the following:

- recording the patient's smoking status
- issuing a final month's supply of NRT or bupropion.

At 3 months and 12 months, use follow-up telephone calls to record the outcome.

Most quit attempts are unsuccessful. It takes an average of three to five attempts before most successful quitters succeed for one year or more, and a failed attempt should be interpreted in that light, with encouragement given to the patient to learn from the experience and consider trying again at a later date.

Prescribing

National Institute for Clinical Excellence (NICE) guidance on prescribing is awaited, but guidelines are available that are broadly similar and widely disseminated.

Attempts to ration prescribing by an assessment of risk are not warranted. The benefits of stopping smoking are very large for anyone who quits. However, indiscriminate prescribing is also unwarranted, and a small number of 'social smokers' may not require pharmacological support.

Perhaps the first step in decision making about whether to prescribe should be based on an assessment of motivation. Motivation is a prerequisite for success, and the pharmacotherapies can only help a motivated patient. Any assessment of motivation is inevitably subjective, but GPs are well placed to make this judgement, aided by their ability to offer continuity of care and their 'premorbid knowledge' of their patients.

Measurement of dependence may be less subjective, but there are still no clear rules about who to prescribe for. The current consensus is that dependence is likely if smokers consume more than 10 cigarettes a day so that the prescription of NRT or bupropion is justified. However, there is no evidence to indicate that there is *no* benefit in individuals who smoke less than this, and it may be a better service to patients to apply this guideline flexibly.

A first principle of prescribing guidelines is the use of abstinent–contingent protocols – in other words, only continuing to prescribe NRT for smokers who have, to date, successfully stopped.

Many patients will resume smoking within 2 weeks, and issuing a month's treatment is wasteful. There is some motivational gain to be had from reassessing the patient with a carbon monoxide measurement soon after the quit date. Patients who are prescribed bupropion will only have set their quit date about 10 days after starting to take the drug, so an initial prescription for 4 weeks' supply may be more appropriate.

In general, the aim should be to offer the smoker the best possible chance of stopping on any and every serious quit attempt.

Nicotine replacement therapy (NRT)

The first NRT product to become available on the UK market was gum. Introduced in 1981, it was initially available on a prescription-only licence. However, the Advisory Committee on Borderline Substances decided that it should not be available on reimbursable NHS prescription, and therefore could only be obtained by private prescription. When 'blacklisting' was introduced in 1985, the gum was automatically added to the list. In 1991, the Medicines Control Agency changed the status of the gum and it became available through pharmacies (under the supervision of a pharmacist) only. In 1993, NRT patches were introduced on the same basis, with a subsequent rapid expansion in the variety of delivery devices. All of them remained blacklisted on the grounds that 'the cost to the NHS if the products were to be supplied on prescription could not be justified at any price likely to be economic to the manufacturer, and that the supply of the product is not considered a priority.'

With the development of specialist smoking cessation services came an opportunity to provide a 1-week supply in exchange for a voucher, but only to smokers referred to the service. GPs remained unable to provide a prescription. This did little to reward the efforts that a successful quitter had made at 1 week, and in effect resulted in the premature withdrawal of a successful treatment. To some extent this over-cautious approach to prescription may have had its foundation in concern about the risks of continued prescriptions being provided in the face of continued smoking. The demonstration of a convincing case for the cost-effectiveness of prescribing NRT in primary care means that it is now available on NHS prescription. Well-implemented and effective guidelines for its use have been developed and applied by both the specialist smoking cessation service and practice-based smoking cessation advisers.

Box 7.4 NRT prescribing guidelines

- Generally only prescribe NRT for those who smoke 10 or more cigarettes daily, but be prepared to be flexible.
- Prescriptions should only be provided for those who are willing to attend smoking cessation support schemes.
- Prescriptions should be contingent upon abstinence – but the occasional slip may be allowable!
- The initial prescription should be for 1 to 2 weeks only.
- Give a repeat prescription thereafter for a further 3 weeks, followed by a further 4 weeks, ideally issued as two prescriptions with confirmation of abstinence in between by carbon monoxide monitoring.
- An 8-week course is sufficient. There is no evidence that a tapered dose is helpful.

The pharmacology and mechanisms of delivery of the range of NRT products available are discussed in detail in Chapter 4. In this section, brief consideration will be given to prescribing information. Other sources of information, particularly the *British National Formulary* and manufacturers' summaries of product characteristics should also be consulted.

The plethora of delivery systems and the range of available doses of NRT reflects the attempt to match an individual smoker's pattern with nicotine replacement therapy (*see* Appendix 3).

The regulatory system is almost certainly over-cautious in its advice about the use of NRT in smokers under 18 years of age, pregnant smokers and smokers with heart disease. Some care is required when considering prescribing NRT for patients with cardiovascular disease or diabetes (in the latter case because the release of catecholamines from the adrenal medulla may impair glucose control; caution is also advised in patients with hyperthyroidism and phaeochromocytoma, for the same reasons), as well as for pregnant and breastfeeding patients. However, nicotine delivered by cigarette is even more harmful due to the addition of associated hydrocarbons and carbon monoxide. Provided that patients are fully informed, perhaps with the additional precaution of providing formal consent, the potential benefits of a quit attempt with NRT far outweigh any risk. When counselling patients in these groups it is worth emphasising that continuing to smoke while using NRT may put them at particular risk of side-effects because of the larger total dose of nicotine. The consequences of weight gain occurring as a result of successfully stopping smoking may need to be tackled later.

- Manufacturers recommend that NRT is contraindicated in patients under 18 years old, but smokers under 18 years of age can certainly be dependent, and there is no sensible reason for denying them NRT.
- There are considerable benefits to stopping smoking in pregnancy, and both Action on Smoking and Health (ASH) and the Royal College of Physicians have recommended that NRT be available. A failed unaided quit attempt should not be a requirement for prescribing NRT.
- Cardiovascular disease risks are increased by nicotine, but in all cases appropriate prescribing of NRT is safer than continuing to smoke, and recent studies of the use of bupropion in cardiovascular disease (excluding stroke) confirm its safety in this group as well.

For a discussion of the variety of delivery systems available and their risks and advantages, *see* Chapter 4.

Some of the specific advantages and problems associated with the range of delivery systems available are outlined below.

Bupropion

Bupropion (Zyban) is an atypical antidepressant, which was made available on prescription as an aid to smoking cessation in the UK in July 2000.

Bupropion has more serious side-effects than NRT, and has tended to be regarded as a second-line drug. Indeed, initial guidelines for prescribing it suggested that it should only be used if a previous serious quit attempt had been made using NRT. However, the limited research on efficacy has suggested that it may have some advantages over NRT, and patients may be better motivated in their desire to try the drug for the first time, or their experience may lead them to prefer it.

Safety scares about the use of bupropion have been reported. A total of 50 sudden deaths have been associated with it in the media and widely misunderstood as having a causal link to it. However, 8 million people have used it worldwide, and the risks are many thousands of times lower than in those who continue to smoke.

Bupropion has a complex pharmacology and inhibits the drug-metabolising enzyme cytochrome P450 2D6, giving it considerable potential to interact with other drugs. Studies suggest that it is well tolerated, although there is a 1 in 1000 dose-dependent risk of seizures. The Medicines Control Agency received 126 reports of seizures in the 419 000 patients who were prescribed bupropion up to May 2001. Around 50% of these patients had predisposing factors that might have precluded the prescription of bupropion if existing guidelines and prescribing advice had been adhered to. The Committee on Safety of Medicines subsequently recommended changes to prescribing practice.

For an account of the side-effects and interactions, the Summary of Product Characteristics (SPC) is available from the manufacturers. Below is a conservative list that was developed for use in a recent study of bupropion in a general practice setting, and which could reasonably form the basis of a pre-prescription checklist for GPs.

Box 7.5 Bupropion

Contraindications

1 Previous hypersensitivity reaction to bupropion.
2 Predisposition to lowered seizure threshold/increased risk of seizures:

- previous head injury
- previous seizure disorder or family history
- brain tumour
- cerebrovascular disease
- alcohol abuse
- severe hepatic cirrhosis
- diabetes treated with oral hypoglycaemics or insulin.

3 Susceptibility to psychotic episodes or panic disorder.
4 History of bipolar disorder or eating disorder.
5 Current pregnancy.
6 Currently breastfeeding.

Cautions: can prescribe, but reduce dose to 150 mg/day.

1 Renal impairment.
2 Mild/moderate hepatic impairment.
3 Elderly.

Co-prescribing: avoid prescribing bupropion if the patient is taking drugs for the above or the following drugs that produce those effects or induce metabolic enzymes.

1   Systemic steroids.
2   Theophyllines.
3   Tricyclics, selective serotonin reuptake inhibitors, monoamine oxidase inhibitors or any other antidepressant.
4   Antipsychotics.
5   Psychoactive drugs, including tranquillizers and hypnotics.
6   Orphenadrine, levodopa or any other drug for Parkinson's disease.
7   Cyclophosphamide/ifosfamide.
8   Carbamezepine, phenobarbitone, valproate, phenytoin or any other anti-epileptic.
9   Appetite suppressants.
10 Beta-blockers.
11 Class 1c anti-arrhythmics – may need dosage adjustment of these drugs; not necessarily contraindicated.

Guidelines for the prescription of bupropion are awaited from the National Institute for Clinical Excellence (NICE).

Box 7.6 shows a suggested protocol in current use.

Box 7.6 Bupropion: guidelines for prescribing

- Previous serious unsuccessful quit attempt using NRT.
- Second courses of bupropion are generally only prescribed after an interval of 6 months and a reassessment of motivation.
- Smoking more than 10 cigarettes daily.
- Only prescribed as part of participation in a smoking cessation scheme.

- Advise against pregnancy and breastfeeding while taking bupropion.
- Treatment is started while the patient is still smoking and a target quit date is set, preferably in the second week.
- The initial dose is 150 mg, to be taken daily for 6 days, increasing on day 7 to 150 mg twice daily.
- There should be an interval of at least 8 hours between successive doses. The maximum total daily dose should not exceed 300 mg.
- Those patients who cannot tolerate the higher dose can be maintained on 150 mg daily.

The course of bupropion is started before the patient's target quit date to allow adequate serum levels to be reached at an initial dose of 150 mg (1 tablet daily) for 6 days followed by 150 mg twice daily for the remainder of the course.

It may be that, as more evidence emerges, combinations of different delivery mechanisms of NRT and bupropion are shown to be more effective than either alone, but at present there is insufficient evidence to recommend this approach.

In their submission to NICE, Action on Smoking and Health (ASH) was strongly and convincingly supportive of the view that both groups of drug should remain available on NHS prescription. ASH concluded that 'failure to treat smoking should be regarded in much the same way as failure to detect and treat pneumonia or other obvious life-threatening conditions' and that 'practitioners who do not offer treatment for tobacco dependence to those in their care are acting negligently.'

The specialist smoking cessation services

Specialist smoking cessation services are now running in all health authorities. They provide more intensive behavioural support to improve the likelihood of success, and they provide training especially for primary care so that each practice has the option of offering on-site support.

Nationally, at present around five smokers per year in an average practice list of 2000 patients use specialist support services together with NRT or bupropion.

The specialist services organise and run groups for smokers trying to quit which are open to all smokers either by referral or directly through local advertising. After an introductory meeting at which the use of NRT and bupropion are discussed (including their risks and side-effects), those who are sufficiently motivated are invited to return for a preparation session and to set a target quit date (TQD) for the following week. NRT or Zyban is recommended. Weekly meetings are held for the first 4 weeks. Request letters for bupropion or NRT prescriptions are taken to the GP for issue. Responsibility for prescribing rests with the GP.

The range of activities of the specialist smoking cessation services includes the following:

- providing telephone support for professionals and the public
- disseminating new information on smoking issues
- supporting network meetings of smoking cessation advisers
- facilitating training
- developing and maintaining specialist smoking cessation services
- giving feedback on monitoring and evaluation data.

The future of the services is rather uncertain. Prescribing budgets have been increased but not ring-fenced, and finances for the specialist services will not be ring-fenced either from April 2002. Services will be commissioned from within primary care, and concerns have been expressed as to whether there will be adequate funding to ensure continuing provision.

Audit

The culture of audit is well established in primary care, and it is as important in developing a smoking cessation programme as in other areas of activity.

The need to collect data across all levels of smoking cessation activity in a uniform manner was considered earlier, and the same requirement applies in developing practice audit. Performing practice audit in ways that allow pooling across the range of services, and comparison between practices, has obvious advantages.

It is probably sensible to start small and begin with simple achievable standards – for example, ensuring that as many patients as possible have a history of smoking status recorded within the previous year.

The Health of the Nation health promotion target, now abandoned, was a smoking history in 80% of the population.

Box 7.7 summarises the development of a practice audit cycle.

Box 7.7 Developing practice audit: an illustration

Aims

1 To increase the accurate and up-to-date recording of the smoking status of patients in the practice.
2 To offer advice and practical support to smokers who wish to stop.
3 To support children and teenagers and encourage them not to start smoking.

Year 1: Setting standards

Objectives

1 To search computer records for the smoking status of all patients over the age of 16 years.
2 To search for a record of smoking status in at-risk groups, including those with a history of coronary heart disease or diabetes.

Outcomes
The results were presented to a meeting of all those in the practice concerned with recording smoking status. The aims of the meeting were as follows:

1 to review and improve the mechanisms for recording smoking status
2 to develop and improve the practice's stop-smoking clinic
3 to set standards for the future recording of smoking status in practice patients.

Disappointment was expressed at the lack of smoking information about patients with coronary heart disease. The new coronary heart disease clinic has only recently started, and the protocol includes a regular review of smoking status. Figures for this should improve.

Data from new patient medical questionnaires about smoking status are not finding their way into the computer record, but entry of these data can be improved without any change to existing systems.

Concern was expressed about the need to record annually 'non-smoker' for those who have never smoked and who are highly unlikely to take up the habit. However, given that we cannot assume no record of smoking is equivalent to non-smoking, it was agreed that it was necessary to continue to do this.

Standards
Agreed at the meeting, these were as follows.

1   Recording:

- 80% of patients aged 16–74 years should have a smoking history recorded within the previous 12 months.
- 90% of patients with a past history of coronary heart disease or diabetes should have a record of smoking status made within the previous 12 months.

2   Cessation activity: 80% of patients prescribed NRT or Zyban should have their smoking status recorded 12 months later.

Year 2: Monitoring performance

Objectives
To search the practice computer records for:

1   smoking-related data to compare the practice's performance against the standards agreed 12 months ago
2   the number of recorded pregnancies over the previous year in which a record of smoking status was made
3   the number of patients with a diagnosis of chronic obstructive pulmonary disease with a record of smoking status within the previous year
4   the numbers of prescriptions for NRT and Zyban within the previous year.

Outcomes
The results were to be presented at a primary healthcare team meeting at which:

1   standards for recording for the succeeding year would be agreed
2   recording interventions would be agreed
3   discussion of further initiatives would take place.

The following points were raised at the meeting:

- The best definition of a patient with chronic obstructive pulmonary disease would be someone attending the practice clinic, as only these patients will definitely have had respiratory function testing. Therefore the standard for recording should be 100% of those attending the COPD clinic.

- Recording when patients had been advised to stop was clinically important in order to avoid unproductive repetition and frustration in consultations with smokers.
- Midwives now have access to the practice computer record system during their clinics, and have agreed to enter smoking-related data.
- Less than 50% of smokers who had made a quit attempt with Zyban or NRT had their status recorded 12 months later. A computer-generated list of contact details for this group of patients would be produced (monthly) on the anniversary of their attempt. The practice smoking cessation adviser would follow up by phone or letter.

Standards

The following standards were agreed at the meeting:

- 90% of patients aged 16–74 years should have a smoking history recorded within the previous 12 months
- 100% of patients with a past history of coronary heart disease, diabetes or COPD should have a record of smoking status made within the previous 12 months
- 100% of patients who had been pregnant within the previous year should have a record of smoking status made.

Cessation activity

- All smokers who have been advised to stop should have the appropriate Read code entered.
- Of those patients prescribed NRT or Zyban, 80% should have their smoking status recorded 12 months later.

Reflection exercises

Exercise 13

Are all of the members of the practice team (including the receptionists and other non-clinical staff) familiar with your practice protocol for the options that are available to help smokers? If not, review your guidelines or protocol at a practice team meeting, and ensure that everyone knows what their roles and responsibilities are.

Undertake an audit of five patients who have been provided with help through the practice's smoking cessation services in the last 12 months. Look back at their medical notes to see how long it took for them to quit. Ascertain whether they have been monitored during a follow-up period, according to your practice protocol.

Make changes to your systems and procedures if your records are inadequate and you do not have follow-up information (e.g. introduce telephone contact after patients have been counselled about stopping smoking or have received pharmacotherapy).

Exercise 14

Do you have a well-established screening programme targeted at high-risk patients in your practice? If not, draft guidelines or a protocol to be agreed with your practice team. If you do have such a programme, undertake an audit of 20 patients with hypertension and see whether their smoking status has been recorded or updated within the last year. If they are smokers, have they received advice about quitting smoking within the last year?

Are your records computerised with appropriate Read coding so that you can conduct audits easily and randomly select patients from a disease register? If not, take 20 consecutive patients with hypertension as they consult you instead.

Now that you have completed this interactive reflection exercise, transfer the information to the empty template of the personal development plan on pages 169–178 if you are working on your own learning plan, or to the practice personal and professional development plan on pages 193–199 if you are working on a practice team learning plan. Don't forget to keep the evidence of your learning in your personal portfolio.

Reference

1 Stapleton J (2001) *Cost-Effectiveness of NHS Smoking Cessation Services.* King's College London Institute of Psychiatry; www.ash.org.uk.

CHAPTER 8

Clinical governance and smoking cessation

Clinical governance is about doing anything and everything required to maximise the quality of healthcare or services provided for, and received by, individual patients or the general population – in this case, people who are at risk of or suffer from smoking-related conditions.[1,2]

We should be able to use clinical governance to improve the delivery of preventive services (e.g. support for smoking cessation) and control of smoking-related conditions (e.g. cardiovascular disease). Clinical governance is inclusive – making quality everyone's business, whether they are a doctor, a nurse or other health professional, a manager, a member of the non-clinical staff or a strategic planner. Everyone in the multidisciplinary healthcare team has a role to play in supporting a person who is trying to stop smoking. Delivering best practice requires sufficient clinical staff who are up to date and relate well to their patients, working with efficient systems and procedures that are patient friendly.

Components of clinical governance[2]

The components of clinical governance are not new. However, bringing them together under the banner of clinical governance and introducing more explicit accountability for performance is a new style of working.

The following 14 themes are core components of professional and service development which together form a comprehensive approach to providing high-quality healthcare services and clinical governance.[2] These are illustrated in Figure 8.1.

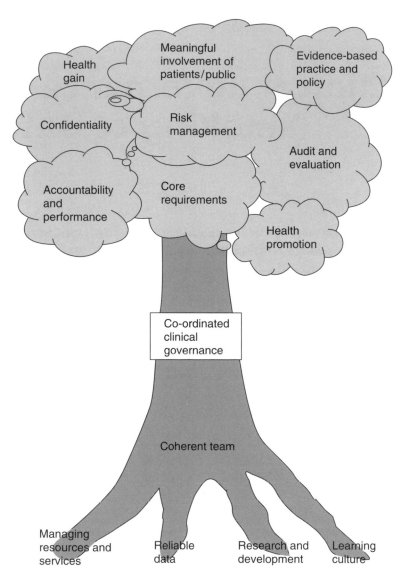

Figure 8.1: 'Routes' and branches of clinical governance.

If you interweave these 14 components into your individual and workplace-based personal and professional development plans, you will have addressed the requirements for clinical governance at the same time.

1 *Learning culture*: for patients and staff in a practice or primary care organisation (PCO) or in secondary care.
2 *Research and development culture*: in the practice or throughout the health service.

3 *Reliable and accurate data*: in the practice, and across the primary care organisation and the NHS as a seamless whole.

4 *Well-managed resources and services*: as individuals, as a practice, across the NHS and in conjunction with other organisations.

5 *Coherent teamwork*: well-integrated teams within a practice, including attached staff.

6 *Meaningful involvement of patients and the public*: including those with smoking-related conditions such as cardiovascular disease, those who care for them and the general population.

7 *Health gain*: from improving the health of patients and staff as a result of stopping smoking.

8 *Confidentiality*: of information at the reception desk, in consultations, in medical notes, between practitioners and with regard to the outside world.

9 *Evidence-based practice and policy*: applying it in practice, in the district and across the NHS.

10 *Accountability and performance*: for standards, performance of individuals and the practice – to the public and those in authority.

11 *Core requirements*: good fit with skill mix and whether individuals are competent to do their jobs; communication, work-force numbers and morale.

12 *Health promotion*: for patients, the public, your staff and colleagues – either opportunistic or by targeting those at risk.

13 *Audit and evaluation*: for instance, of the extent to which individuals and practice teams adhere to best practice in identifying and advising patients who smoke tobacco.

14 *Risk management*: being competent to detect those at risk, reducing risks and probability of ill health, and following up high-risk patients.

The challenges to delivering clinical governance

Delivering high-quality healthcare, with guaranteed minimum standards of care at all times, is a major challenge. At present the quality of healthcare is patchy and variable. We are not very good at detecting under-performance and rectifying it at an early stage. The small number of clinicians who do under-perform exert a disproportionately large effect on the public's confidence. Causes of under-performance in an individual might be a result of a lack of knowledge or skills, poor attitudes or ill health or a lack of resources. Poor management is nearly always a contributory reason for inadequate clinical services.

We need to understand why variation exists and explore ways of reducing inequalities. Variation in the quality of healthcare provided is common, whether it is between different practices in the same locality, between staff of the same discipline working in the same practice or unit, or between care given to some groups of the population rather than others.

Clinical governance offers a co-ordinated approach to overcoming these areas of risk.[3] The complex cultural change that will be required to deliver uniformly excellent care is immense. We need to develop measurable outcomes that professionals, patients and the public consider to be relevant and meaningful. Then we can assess the progress made, through implementing clinical governance, in the milestones and targets set out in national guidance for managing coronary heart disease and smoking cessation.

Having an up-to-date record describing whether and which patients smoke can act as a tracer condition for a clinical governance programme. Applying best practice when recording patients' smoking status requires a well-established infrastructure (good IT systems and a patient register), links to disease registers such as those for asthma, diabetes and coronary heart disease, evidence-based protocols, monitoring systems, competent staff and multidisciplinary teamwork.

Learning culture

Education and training programmes should be relevant to service needs, whether at organisational or individual levels. Continuing professional development (CPD) programmes need to meet both the learning needs of individual health professionals and the wider service development needs of the NHS. You should no longer opt for CPD activities according to what you *want* to do, but rather according to what you *need* to do. Clinical governance underpins professional and service development.

> **Individual personal development plans**
> will feed into a
> **workplace- or practice-based personal and
> professional development plan**
> that will feed into
> **the primary care organisation's business plan**
> all of which are
> **underpinned by clinical governance.**[4]

Multidisciplinary learning helps the team to work closely to provide well co-ordinated multidisciplinary care. An in-house educational meeting provides an opportunity to agree a common approach, such as that of the 'six As' (*see* Chapter 6).

1 *Ask* about smoking on a regular basis.
2 *Advise* current smokers about the value of stopping.
3 *Assess* their motivation to stop.
4 *Assist* the motivated smoker in stopping.
5 *Arrange* follow-up visits.
6 *Audit* what has been achieved.[5]

Applying research and development in practice

The findings of the many thousands of research papers about smoking and smoking-related conditions that are published in reputable journals each year are rarely applied in practice. This is because few health professionals or managers read such journals regularly, so they are not aware of the research findings. Most practice teams do not have a system for reviewing important research papers and translating that review into practical action. The primary care organisation might help by relaying important new evidence to its constituent practices or the general public. Agreeing on local disease templates (e.g. for coronary heart disease) backed by resources should enable change to occur.

> Incorporating research-based evidence into everyday practice should promote policies on effective working, improve quality and contribute to a clinical governance culture.

Research increases our understanding of the reasons why people smoke and the effects of smoking on their health and well-being. It also throws more light on the most effective interventions for helping people to stop smoking.

A postal survey of around 1000 people in one general practice found that where smokers attributed their respiratory symptoms to smoking they were eight times more likely to believe that their health would improve if they stopped smoking, and six times more likely to intend to stop smoking.[6]

Reliable and accurate data

Clinicians, patients and administrators need access to reliable and accurate data. Set standards for a general practice to:

- keep records in chronological order
- summarise medical records (within a specified time period for records of new patients)
- review dates for checks on smoking status for high-risk patient groups, with audit in place to monitor whether standards are adhered to, and to plan for under-performance if necessary
- use computers for diagnostic recording – agree Read codes for classifying smoking status
- record information from external sources (hospital and other organisations) that is relevant to individual patients or practice.

Keep good written records of policies and audits that relate to smoking status and smoking-related conditions in the practice. An inspection at any time should show what audits have been undertaken and when, the changes in practice organisation that followed, the extent of staff training undertaken, and the future programme of monitoring.

There is still a great deal of resistance to full computerisation in practice teams. Ten ways to increase your team's enthusiasm for developing your IT infrastructure are listed below.[7]

1 Start by considering your needs, not the technology.
2 Invest heavily in training for clinicians as well as IT staff.
3 Involve clinicians in all IT decisions.
4 Regard technology as a means to an end.

5 Use proper project management techniques.
6 Use the best IT staff you can.
7 Ensure that the IT solution delivers better patient care and clinical benefits.
8 Ensure that the suppliers deliver what is promised.
9 Adopt recommended solutions across the primary care organisation (PCO) to minimise compatibility problems.
10 Adopt a PCO-wide coding policy.

There will be little progress in improving the quality of data across a primary care organisation or trust unless staff have been adequately trained in using computers and recording patient-related data. The Audit Commission has published a self-evaluation checklist for primary care organisations and trusts.[8] It contains useful suggestions for challenging the quality of patient-based information across a trust or a practice or workplace team. The testing and monitoring of these standards should form the basis of a series of worthwhile audits. Any healthcare employers can self-evaluate their approach by asking themselves the following questions.[8]

- What percentage of staff have received training in the use of information systems?
- What form did the training take?
- To what extent does the training and development in the use of information systems include training in data quality?
- In what ways does the PCO/trust/practice make use of patient-based information (e.g. the smoking status of patients)?

Well-managed resources and services

The things you need to achieve best practice should be in the right place at the right time and working correctly every time.
  Set standards in your practice or workplace for:

- access to premises and availability of services for people with special needs (e.g. those with disability due to heart disease or stroke)
- provision of routine and urgent appointments (e.g. for those with coronary heart disease)
- access to and provision for smoking cessation services
- proactive monitoring of smoking status and changes in smoking habits after an intervention such as drug treatment

- alternatives to face-to-face consultations
- consultation length.

Systems should be designed to prevent and detect errors. Therefore it is important to keep systems simple and sensible, and to inform everyone how those systems operate, so that they are less likely to bypass a system or make errors. Sort out good systems for the follow-up of patients with smoking-related conditions such as coronary heart disease and stroke.

Coherent teamwork

Teams do produce better patient care than single practitioners operating in a fragmented way. Effective teams make the most of the different contributions of individual clinical disciplines in delivering patient care. The characteristics of effective teams are:

- shared ownership of a common purpose
- clear goals for the contribution that each discipline makes
- open communication between team members
- opportunities for team members to enhance their skills.

A team approach helps different team members to adopt an evidence-based approach to patient care, by having to justify their approach to the rest of the team.[9] With smoking cessation, teamwork between practice team members is particularly important, so that all are giving consistent messages about the risks of smoking and the interventions offered by the practice. Pharmacists should work closely with practice teams, especially if they are providing 'stop smoking' initiatives.

Meaningful involvement of patients and the public

Patients or carers, non-users of services, the local community, particular subgroups of the population or the general public will all have useful feedback and views. For example, ask for their views about the quality or type of healthcare on offer, the planning of future services, your systems, or how to locate services closer to the patient.

> The British Heart Foundation involves people who are suffering from cardiovascular problems in the preparation of their educational literature for patients, so that it is appropriate for individuals' needs and preferences.

The aims of user involvement and public participation include better outcomes of individual care and the health of the population, more locally responsive services and greater ownership of health services.[10] Those planning the services should develop a better understanding of why and how local services need to be changed. For example, you might want to consult the public and health professionals about the closure of a community hospital, without which those with chronic smoking-related conditions such as coronary heart disease may have to travel further for their care.

Interactive information may work well in involving patients in their own healthcare by forcing them to confront the reasons why they should give up smoking cigarettes. The interactive website www.givingupsmoking.co.uk is a good example of a resource that may be helpful.

You might consider asking several ex-smokers whether any of the services or advice that you have provided made a difference to their giving up smoking. Ask them how you could improve your services or information giving – and feed that back to the rest of the practice team.

Health gain

Smoking is the single greatest cause of preventable illness and premature death in the UK. About half of all lifelong smokers will die of smoking-related diseases.[5]

The two general approaches to improving health are the 'population' approach, which focuses on measures to improve health through the community, and the 'high-risk' approach, which focuses on vulnerable individuals who are at high risk of the condition or hazard.

The population strategy aims to shift the whole distribution of a risk factor in a favourable direction.[11] However, the 'prevention paradox' means that preventive actions that greatly benefit the population as a whole may bring only small benefits for individuals.

> Changing the population distribution of a risk factor is better than targeting people who are at high risk.[11]

The high-risk approach aims to detect people at high risk of disease and to lower their risk by providing treatment. We generally use a targeted approach in primary care to identify patients who are at risk or whose coronary heart disease is currently undiagnosed, rather than a population-based approach.

> Stopping smoking can reduce the rate of decline in lung function in most patients with chronic obstructive pulmonary disease, and can improve the survival rate. Smoking cessation does not restore lung function that has already been lost.[12]

The two approaches are not mutually exclusive, and they often need to be combined with legislation and community action. Health goals include the following:

- a good quality of life
- avoiding premature death
- equal opportunities for health.

Confidentiality

Confidentiality is a component of clinical governance that is often overlooked. Experienced health professionals and managers may assume that junior or new staff know all about confidentiality, and of course they may not. There are many difficult situations in the NHS where one person asks for information about another's medical condition. For example, it is not always clear-cut whether test results should be given to or withheld from someone else enquiring on the patient's behalf if the patient is vulnerable in some way (e.g. affected by a severe stroke).

The Caldicott Committee Report describes the following principles of good practice to safeguard confidentiality when information is being used for non-clinical purposes.[13]

- Justify the purpose.
- Do not use patient-identifiable information unless it is absolutely necessary to do so.
- Use the minimum necessary patient-identifiable information.
- Access to patient-identifiable information should be on a strict need-to-know basis.

- Everyone with access to patient-identifiable information should be aware of his or her responsibilities.

A practice nurse was keen to start up groups to help people to stop smoking. She proposed sending letters to all those whose personal history included a record that they smoked. When her project was discussed at the practice meeting, she was upset to realise that she had not considered the implications of using the information given for one purpose for another. The practice manager was able to point out that she might be fielding a complaint if someone objected to the use of their information in this way, especially if it revealed information that had been hidden from other members of the family. It was decided to send a general mailing inviting anyone who smoked and was interested in the practice nurse's group work to send back a reply slip.

Evidence-based culture: policy and practice

The key features determining whether or not local guidelines worked in one initiative[14] were as follows.

- There was multidisciplinary involvement in drawing them up.
- A systematic review of the literature underpinned the guidelines, with graded recommendations for best practice linked to the evidence.
- There was ownership at both national and local levels.
- A local implementation plan ensured that the needs for resources, time, staff, education and training were foreseen, met and supported.
- Plans were made to sustain the guidelines – which were user friendly and could be modified to suit individual practitioners and patients.

There are several systems for grading evidence. A classification[15] that is often quoted gives the strength of evidence as shown in Box 8.1.

Box 8.1 Strength of evidence

Type I: Strong evidence from at least one systematic review of multiple well-designed randomised controlled trials (RCTs).

Type II: Strong evidence from at least one properly designed randomised controlled trial of appropriate size.

Type III: Evidence from well-designed trials without randomisation, single group pre–post, cohort, time-series or matched case–control studies.

Type IV: Evidence from well-designed non-experimental studies from more than one centre or research group.

Type V: The opinions of respected authorities, based on clinical evidence, descriptive studies or reports of expert committees.

Other categories of evidence are listed in the compendium of the best available evidence for effective healthcare. *Clinical Evidence,*[16] which is updated every six months. This categorisation of evidence is perhaps more useful to the health professional in everyday work (*see* Box 8.2).

Box 8.2

Beneficial: Interventions whose effectiveness has been shown by clear evidence from controlled trials.

Likely to be beneficial: Interventions for which effectiveness is less well established than for those listed under 'beneficial'.

Trade-off between benefits and harms: Interventions for which clinicians and patients should weigh up the beneficial and harmful effects according to individual circumstances and priorities.

Unknown effectiveness: Interventions for which there are currently insufficient data, or data of inadequate quality (this includes interventions that are widely accepted as beneficial but which have never been formally tested in randomised control trials (RCTs), often because the latter would be regarded as unethical).

Unlikely to be beneficial: Interventions for which lack of effectiveness is less well established than for those listed under 'likely to be ineffective or harmful'.

Likely to be ineffective or harmful: Interventions whose ineffectiveness or harmfulness has been demonstrated by clear evidence.

One study of national smoking cessation guidelines found four such guidelines written in English. The authors reported that systematic reviews commonly underpinned the recommendations in these guidelines on smoking cessation. They called for greater international collaboration in sharing research resources that would allow guideline developers to access the most recent evidence in order to reduce the costs and effort associated with further local guideline development.[17]

Accountability and performance

Health professionals may not always realise that they are accountable to others from outside their own professions, especially if they have self-employed status, as do GPs, pharmacists and dentists. However, in fact they are accountable to:

- the general public
- their profession – to maintain the standards of knowledge and skills of the profession as a whole
- the Government – and employer, who expect high standards of healthcare from the work-force.

It is possible to identify and rectify under-performance at an early stage by, for example:

- regular appraisals (at least annually) linked to clinical governance and personal development plans; appraisals should be supportive meetings, but they need a mechanism for dealing with under-performance if it crops up
- detecting those who have significant health problems, and referring them for help
- systematic audit that distinguishes an individual's performance from the overall performance of the practice team
- an open learning culture in which team members are discouraged from covering up colleagues' inadequacies, so that problems can be resolved at an early stage.

Clinicians may regard the NHS performance assessment framework as a management tool that is not particularly relevant to their clinical practice. However, it does reinforce a clinical governance culture whereby good clinical and organisational management have a symbiotic relationship.

> The NHS performance assessment framework has six components, namely health improvement, fair access, efficiency, effective delivery of appropriate care, user/carer experience and health outcomes.

Health promotion

Good-quality information will help people who smoke to make choices about their smoking habit and other health-related behaviour, such as their diet and level of physical activity. Simple brief advice about stopping smoking, given by doctors or nurses to patients who smoke during their routine care, increases the likelihood of long-term smoking cessation by more than 50%.[5]

Nicotine replacement therapy and buproprion nearly double the success rates of smoking cessation intervention compared with placebo (*see* Chapter 4). The website www.right-time.co.uk gives patients who have been prescribed buproprion motivational support online as they attempt to stop smoking. The site includes health-promoting techniques such as a calendar to record success, an action planner with tips on avoiding temptation to resume smoking, a health benefits chart to reinforce the health advantages of being a non-smoker, and an accessible helpline.

> Smoking cessation services have been targeted at the 26 Health Action Zones in England and their disadvantaged populations. Most have concentrated on young people and pregnant women as priority groups to limit the harmful effects of smoking on future generations.[18]

In one study of young people's attitudes to smoking,[19] over 75% of those aged 16–24 years who were surveyed declared that they would not smoke if they had their time over again. Most smokers overestimated the likelihood of stopping smoking in the future, and greatly underestimated how long it was likely to take to become and stay an ex-smoker. The authors of the study describe this mismatch between smokers' expectations about how easy and quick they believe it will be to stop smoking, and the likelihood of stopping smoking in reality, as the 'delusion gap'.

The state of readiness to change is the basis of one popular approach to understanding human behaviour. It is important for doctors and nurses to know where smokers are in the 'cycle of change', so that they can inform, motivate and support them appropriately.[20] During the 'pre-contemplation' stage, a person is content to be smoking and is not considering taking action to quit. In the 'contemplation' stage, the person is dissatisfied with being a smoker and is thinking about giving up smoking. A person in the 'preparation' stage is making serious plans to stop smoking. Hopefully they will then move into the 'action' stage and attempt to stop smoking. During the 'maintenance' stage, the person tries not to resume smoking. The 'relapse' stage occurs if they start smoking again despite their best endeavours to remain an ex-smoker.

Audit and evaluation

Audit will probably be the method you think of first for assessing how well you are doing and what it is you need to learn.

You might look at the extent to which you are adhering to the primary care organisation's or practice's protocol for tackling smoking (*see* Appendix 4) (e.g. whether you are giving consistent advice to all smokers and prescribing pharmacotherapies appropriately). For example, you could check that bupropion has not been prescribed for any patients for whom it is contraindicated. These patients would be those recorded as having a previous history of seizures, bulimia or anorexia nervosa, or those taking other medications that lower their seizure threshold (e.g. antipsychotic or antidepressant drugs, theophylline or systemic steroids).

You could look at the quality of data that everyone in your organisation is collecting about patients, using smoking status as an indicator of performance because it is relevant to a wide range of clinical conditions. For instance, to what extent is the trust, primary care organisation or practice using comparative information to identify areas of variation that may be due to data quality?[8] For example, are all GPs and nurses recording the smoking status of patients who are consulting them consistently? Are all members of staff using the same computer codes, to classify smoking status?

Core requirements

You cannot deliver clinical governance without well-trained and competent staff, the right skill mix of staff, and a safe and comfortable working environment.

There is accumulating evidence that helping people to stop smoking according to best practice is cost-effective, but further research is still needed to investigate the relative cost-effectiveness of different interventions.

The cost of the smoking cessation services run in England between April 2000 and March 2001 is estimated to have been £21.4 million. This involved 500 dedicated staff helping 127 000 smokers set a date to quit smoking. The cost-effectiveness of the new smoking cessation services has been calculated from these figures. They are just over £600 per life-year gained for treated smokers aged 35–44 years, and £750 for those aged 45–54 years.[21] The cost-effectiveness of smoking cessation services compares favourably with that of statin therapies.

There is real concern that resources should be ring-fenced at national level in the long term. Smoking cessation is a high priority, and the newly established smoking cessation services should be funded appropriately.

The core requirements for the NHS are part of a clinical governance culture in relation to the following:

- *partnership*: working together across the NHS to ensure the best possible care
- *performance*: acting to review and deliver higher standards of healthcare
- *the professions and wider work-force*: breaking down barriers between different disciplines (e.g. through multidisciplinary team-work between GPs and nurses with pharmacists and other independent contractors)
- *patient care*: access, convenient services and empowerment to take a full part in decision making about their own medical care and in planning and providing health services in general
- *prevention*: promoting healthy living across all sections of society, tackling variations in care, and encouraging people to take responsibility for their own health (e.g. by stopping smoking and remaining non-smokers).

Nurse-led smoking cessation group
One practice that received recognition as Beacon status for their SmokeStop sessions adopted a small-group approach to smoking cessation rather than providing individual consultations. The practice reported that 80% of the 140 patients who attended the sessions stopped smoking during the course of six sessions for varying periods of time, and 15% were not smoking three months after their quit day.[22]

Risk management

People may underestimate relative risks as applied to themselves and their own behaviour. For example, many smokers accept the relationship between smoking tobacco and disease, but do not believe that they personally are at risk. People usually have a reasonable idea of the *relative risks* of various activities and behaviours, although their personal estimates of the *magnitude* of risks tend to be biased – small probabilities are often over-estimated, and high probabilities are often under-estimated.[3]

Risk management in general practice mainly centres on assessing the probability that potential or actual hazards will give rise to harm. Consider how bad the risk is, how likely the risk is, when the risk will occur, if ever, and how certain you are of estimates about the risks. This applies equally whether the risk is an environmental or organisational one in the practice, or a clinical risk.

Communicating and managing risks on an individual basis with patients depends on finding ways to explain those risks and elicit people's values and preferences. They can then make decisions themselves either to take risks or to choose between alternatives that involve different risks and benefits.

Reflection exercise

Exercise 15

Review and plan your management of patients who smoke. Think how you might integrate the 14 components of clinical governance into your personal development plan or your practice personal and professional development plan. Examples are given for each component listed below. Complete this yourself from your own perspective.

- *Establishing a learning culture*: e.g. informal discussion between GPs, nurses and a community pharmacist about how the practice protocol for smoking cessation and hypertension guidelines interrelate.
- *Managing resources and services*: e.g. review the roles and responsibilities of members of the practice team and attached staff with regard to helping someone to stop smoking after they have had a myocardial infarction.
- *Establishing a research and development culture*: e.g. among the practice team share findings in key research papers on best practice for intervening to stop smoking.
- *Reliable and accurate data*: e.g. keep electronic records (both individual and team) so that everyone uses the same Read codes for smoking status and enters data consistently. Any audit exercises can be repeated the next year and the results compared.
- *Evidence-based practice and policy*: e.g. update your evidence-based protocol for smoking cessation in the practice.
- *Confidentiality*: e.g. check that everyone is adhering to your agreed code of practice for giving results or advice at the reception desk.
- *Health gain*: e.g. target those patients who smoke who have diabetes and/or coronary heart disease, in order to make significant efforts to reduce their risk factors.
- *Coherent team*: e.g. communicate new systems for classifying smoking status to the rest of your practice team.
- *Audit and evaluation*: e.g. undertake a significant event audit and act on the findings to improve the quality of an aspect of care given to patients with smoking-related conditions.
- *Meaningful involvement of patients and the public*: e.g. listen to and act on the comments of those patients who smoke as you try to engage them in making difficult decisions to stop smoking.
- *Health promotion*: e.g. obtain or write literature promoting the benefits of stopping smoking.
- *Risk management*: e.g. establish systems and procedures to identify patients with increased risks of developing smoking-related conditions.
- *Accountability and performance*: e.g. keep good records of smokers as they consult the doctor or nurse, to demonstrate that they have received opportunistic to stop smoking.
- *Core requirements*: e.g. agree roles and responsibilities in the

practice team, such as GP referral to the nurse for help with smoking cessation; train receptionists so that they know the full range of help available to those who want to quit smoking.

References

1 Lilley R (1999) *Making Sense of Clinical Governance.* Radcliffe Medical Press, Oxford.

2 Chambers R and Wakley G (2000) *Making Clinical Governance Work for You.* Radcliffe Medical Press, Oxford.

3 Mohanna K and Chambers R (2001) *Risk Matters: communicating risk, clinical risk management.* Radcliffe Medical Press, Oxford.

4 Wakley G, Chambers R and Field S (2000) *Continuing Professional Development: making it happen.* Radcliffe Medical Press, Oxford.

5 British Heart Foundation (2001) *Stopping Smoking: evidence-based guidance.* Factfile 8/2001. British Heart Foundation, London.

6 Walters N and Coleman T (2002) Comparison of the smoking behaviour and attitudes of smokers who attribute respiratory symptoms to smoking with those who do not. *Br J Gen Pract.* **52**: 132–4.

7 Gillies A (2000) *Information and IT for Primary Care.* Radcliffe Medical Press, Oxford.

8 Audit Commission (2002) *Data Remember. Improving the quality of patient-based information in the NHS.* Audit Commission, London.

9 Miller C, Ross N and Freeman M (1999) *Shared Learning and Clinical Teamwork: new directions in education and multiprofessional practice.* English National Board for Nursing, Midwifery and Health Visiting, University of Brighton, Brighton.

10 Chambers R (2000) *Involving Patients and the Public. How to do it better.* Radcliffe Medical Press, Oxford.

11 Hofman A and Vandenbroucke JP (1992) Geoffrey Rose's big idea. Changing the population distribution of a risk factor is better than targeting people at high risk. *BMJ.* **305**: 1519–20.

12 Pelkonen M, Notkola IL, Tukiainen H, Tervahauta M, Tuomilehto J and Nissinen A (2001) Smoking cessation, decline in pulmonary function and total mortality: a 30-year follow-up study among the Finnish Cohort of the Seven Countries Study. *Thorax.* **56**: 703–7.

13 Department of Health (1997) Report of the review of patient-identifiable information. In: *The Caldicott Committee Report.* Department of Health, London.

14 Donald P (2000) Promoting local ownership of guidelines. *Guidelines Pract.* **3**: 17.

15 Muir Gray JA (1997) *Evidence-Based Healthcare.* Churchill Livingstone, Edinburgh.

16 Barton S (ed.) (2001) *Clinical Evidence. Issue 5.* BMJ Publishing Group, London.

17 Silagy CA, Stead LF and Lancaster T (2001) Use of systematic reviews in clinical practice guidelines: case study of smoking cessation. *BMJ.* **323**: 833–6.

18 Department of Health (2000) *Statistics on Smoking Cessation Services in Health Action Zones: England, April 1999 to March 2000.* Statistical Press Release. Department of Health, London.

19 Jarvis M, McIntyre D and Bates C (2002) Efforts must take into account smokers' disillusionment with smoking and their delusions about stopping (letter). *BMJ.* **324**: 608.

20 Prochaska JO, DiClemente CD and Norcross J (1992) In search of how people change. *Am Psychol.* **47**: 1102–14.

21 Raw M, McNeill A, Watt J *et al.* (2001) National smoking cessation services at risk. *BMJ.* **323**: 1140–41.

22 Russ P (2001) Nurse-led smoking cessation group proves successful. *Guidelines Pract.* **4**: 41–51.

CHAPTER 9

Draw up and apply your personal development plan

A personal development plan (PDP) on the management of smoking cessation could supplement a practice personal and professional development plan (PPDP) (*see* Chapter 10) on cardiovascular disease[1] or learning about other more general health promotion activities.[2] So we have included a worked example of a PDP focused around the management of smoking cessation in your own workplace or practice on pages 182–192.

The example given is very comprehensive and you may not want to include so much in your own PDP. You might include different topics and educational activities, because your needs and circumstances are different from the example practitioner here. You might want to spend half of your available time on this topic and the rest on other priority subjects, such as those in the National Service Frameworks, or topics from your local Health Improvement and Modernisation Plan.

You will need to involve your colleagues and workplace team in anything that you propose, including in your own PDP. Some suggestions are included in the example. Discuss it too with your education and clinical governance leads in your own workplace. They will be able to help you focus on achievable aims and objectives as well and point out any gaps you might not have thought about. Your PDP will need to feed into the practice or workplace development plans as well – so consult as widely as possible before you start. Keep it simple too, so that after a year you will be able to measure some progress. You can then build on that, or change focus for a while, in subsequent years.

Transfer the information about your learning needs from any of the reflection exercises at the end of the chapters that are relevant to you, and that you have completed, to the empty PDP template that follows on pages 169–178. The reflection exercises that you decide to select will depend on the focus of your PDP – as in the worked example here – or on other facets of smoking cessation or smoking-related disease.

The conclusions you have made at the end of each exercise will feature in your PDP's action plan. Some more ideas about the preliminary information you should be gathering for your PDP are given in the boxes of the template.

Worked example of a personal development plan: the management of smoking cessation

Who chose the topic?

It might be your own choice, or that of the team in which you work who think that you should have additional skills in the management of smoking cessation.

Why is the topic a priority?

(i) A personal or professional priority? You may have chosen the management of smoking cessation, seeing a need for it yourself or as an inevitable development in your work. You may have agreed as part of your work development, or as a requirement of a change in work duties or responsibilities. You may have volunteered after development in the management of smoking cessation was identified as a practice or PCO or trust need.

(ii) A practice or workplace priority? The practice may have a need for an in-house expert to provide best practice and reduce costs. Perhaps the practice has identified that the recording of smoking in records is lower than average, or that local need for smoking cessation is higher than average. You may have received a complaint that you did nothing about someone's smoking and that he has now had an amputation because of vascular disease, or a patient of yours may have been the subject of a significant incident analysis. A different skill mix in the practice (e.g. the nurse who did this before has left) may have increased the need for personal expertise in the management of smoking cessation.

(iii) A district priority? The PCO or trust may need a local expert to provide guidelines and services. The PCO may have identified a need to reconsider how services are provided. They may be concerned about

high referral rates to secondary care, or high levels of respiratory illness or cardiovascular events in the area.

(iv) A national priority? The reduction of smoking, and prevention of illnesses associated with, or promoted by, smoking, are important national priorities.

Who will be included in your personal development plan?

You might like to find others who want to increase their skills. Working together, or as a cascade of learning from each other, makes learning more cost-effective and you can set consistent standards of care. Learning skills and then passing them on makes for more effective learning for you too.

Everyone needs to have the opportunity – reception staff, practice manager, secretaries, *all* the health professionals and anyone who uses your premises might benefit from learning about the management of smoking cessation. Disseminating basic information may reduce the workload of health professionals. Remember confidentiality and security issues.

You may want to consider training as a PCO or trust activity to ensure consistency, to exchange skills and to reduce costs. Bringing in outside experts then becomes more cost-effective and training can be tailored to the particular needs of the learning group.

What baseline information will you collect and how?

Ask the practice manager or secretary, or the clinical tutor at the PCO or trust, or the local health promotion department, for details of training available. If you are already Internet connected, you can search for other, more distant, information yourself. If you use external smoking cessation groups or facilitators, ask them for feedback on your referrals – how appropriate they are, how you might modify your management before referral, etc.

You need to know what is being done at present, so set up an audit of your present management. Discover the number of patients recorded as smokers in your practice, and in other practices in your PCO, and compare this with national standards. Establish what provision is already available for the various methods of smoking cessation and, if you can, the numbers of people using the services at present.

Look up guidelines used or advised by other people. Useful resources include the publication *Guidelines in Practice* or the website e-guidelines.[3]

Find out what is in the pipeline for the immediate and long-term future development of the management of smoking cessation in your area.

How will you identify your learning needs?

Amongst other methods you might want to do a SWOT analysis for yourself and with your team:

- *Strengths*: Enthusiasm. An interest in smoking cessation. Willingness to go on learning. Good communication skills and inter-professional relationships to enable inter-disciplinary working. Organisational skills, teaching skills and research skills to provide a resource for the management of smoking cessation. The practice or workplace has sufficient spare capacity for quality improvements and is able to provide a resource for the PCO or trust.
- *Opportunities*: A contact in smoking cessation services for the locality. An individual with skills in the management of smoking cessation, who is enthusiastic to pass on his or her newly acquired knowledge. Expertise at evaluating interventions is available on which you can build to improve professional proficiency. You have decided to develop expertise in the provision of best smoking cessation.
- *Weaknesses and threats*: Deficiencies in equipment, time for carrying out services and in the availability of training. Too many other guidelines and increasing numbers of National Service Framework requirements or other national guidance for the practice team to meet. Other commitments, antagonism or lack of support from others, both inside the practice team and from other practices, and outside the practice from secondary and community services.

You might include a survey of the expertise available in your PCO or trust and elsewhere, and list the present competencies of other staff. What skills and services are accessible inside and outside your own workplace?

What are the learning needs of the practice or workplace and how do they match your needs?

The prioritising exercise should have already given you some information. Consider inviting people to give their concerns and opinions at a practice team meeting or ask another member of staff to organise it. The practice manager could ask the practice team to complete a checklist of their own needs and wishes for the management of smoking cessation, and what they would like from others. The clinical governance lead or development officer of the PCO or trust could do the same for the district.

One staff member might wish to specialise and become an expert in the management of smoking cessation. Does that fit with the requirements of the workplace (or PCO)? Would it be more cost-effective to use that expertise from another practice, workplace or from the existing community services?

A GP might wish to become the GP with a special interest for the PCO, or work in a community clinic or as a clinical assistant in secondary care. What implications does that have for the practice in terms of cover for clinical sessions?

A practice nurse might wish to gain expertise in, and take over much of the work connected with, smoking cessation for patients referred to her from other team members. What implications does that have for her other workload?

You might find that your local community service wishes to take over more of the smoking cessation services and provide a resource for the whole area. Does this have implications for your budget and workload?

You might wish to employ someone with special expertise to supplement what is available within the practice, or provide space for someone to work independently at your practice. What does that mean for your patients and can you recommend that patients attend? Who will pay for the service, and will it make a difference to the income for the practice or department? Will it be independent or managed by the practice or the PCO/trust? Will you need to make alterations to the layout of your premises, or the equipment used? How will that be financed? Do you know what their qualifications mean and what level of service they might be expected to provide?

You might like the PCO to purchase, or arrange to use independently, services at a local clinic for the provision of particular methods of smoking cessation. You may want to provide smoking cessation to all-comers. This requires negotiation with other practices to make sure that they do not feel that you are trying to poach their patients, and negotiation about who is going to pay for the services provided.

Is there any patient or public input to your personal development plan?

You may well have some local experts who could help the practice. Think about how you would go about recruiting them and the implications for confidentiality.

Find out what patients think would be useful – ask for feedback, organise a focus group or set up a representative local group.

You could set up evening or Saturday morning sessions or visit schools, youth clubs, working men's clubs or women's groups to publicise what is and will be available and to obtain feedback on the present provision. Think about inviting a well-known local figure to one or two of the sessions to increase the impact and to get some free publicity (let the local paper or TV/radio station know).

Arrange for computer terminals or poster displays giving access to other sources of advice provided by other agencies (libraries, citizens' advice bureau, the Council).

What mechanism(s) will you use to find out the answers in a meaningful way – not just views from the most opinionated or compliant? You may need to think deeply about the reliability of any method, and how representative individual patients are of your whole practice population.[4]

Aims of your personal development plan arising from the preliminary data-gathering exercise

To learn how to:

- identify the needs of the patients
- provide a good service to meet those needs
- ensure confidentiality
- identify when people are ready to change
- increase knowledge about the availability of services among potential users
- be better informed about methods of smoking cessation
- increase your range of skills in providing methods of smoking cessation
- set up forms for automating recording of clinical encounters, management and activity reports, annual report information, etc.
- identify the patients at high risk from their smoking habit
- increase your skills in identifying psychosocial problems linked with smoking habits
- provide good patient leaflets and information
- set up ways of keeping yourself and other staff up-to-date with current thinking and best practice.

How might you integrate the 14 components of clinical governance into your personal development plan focusing on the topic of smoking cessation?[5]

Establishing a learning culture: searching on the National Electronic Library for Medicine (*see* useful websites) for evidence-based procedures and information, collecting published papers and handouts;

disseminating the information throughout the practice team (including attached staff).

Managing resources and services: identify the extra resources that might be required to provide good quality provision; the skill mix required for delivering smoking cessation; the implications for other services and resources if staff are to add new services to their present roles.

Establishing a research and development culture: set up an automatic information gathering service for articles about provision and management of smoking cessation services on a website; do a before and after study of smoking cessation services in the workplace and PCO or trust.

Reliable and accurate data: enter data once, enter data consistently and correctly; be able to retrieve it for a variety of uses; and be able to compare the data with others.

Evidence-based practice and policy: find out what has worked elsewhere, and how well proven are the interventions you use.

Confidentiality: ensure that the data is protected against unauthorised access and not passed to others without knowing the degree of confidentiality it will be given. Communicate the importance given to confidentiality so that all staff and patients are aware of the rules. Make sure that patients' informed consent is obtained before any named data is given to others.

Health gain: the provision of good quality smoking cessation advice helps to prevent illness and premature death and the social consequences of these.

Coherent team: everyone in the practice team needs to know best practice for the management of smoking cessation.

Audit and evaluation: follow the management of specific methods of smoking cessation; learn to search and audit management and incidents in a multiplicity of ways.

Meaningful involvement of patients and the public: interactive sessions with patients and the public to inform them about, and show ways of providing, smoking cessation; information from leaflets, computer programs, posters.

Health promotion: target health promotion with specific reminders on-screen or select specific groups for action, e.g. those with cardiovascular disease or diabetes, antenatal patients or young women on oral contraceptives.

Risk management: ensure up-to-date records on incidents in the practice; surveys of equipment; surveys of best (or poor) working practices.

Accountability and performance: monitor before and after interventions; reward and celebrate good practice and suggestions.

Core requirements: could you work out a different skill mix in your practice team to provide better provision and management of smoking cessation?

Action learning plan

Who is involved? All identified staff who need to learn about the management of smoking cessation with you.

Where? Identify the sites at which training and learning will take place.

Timetabled action. Start date . . .

By 3 months: preliminary data gathered and staff involved identified.
- Skills that are already present (in the practice, in the PCO or trust, in the community, etc.).
- Equipment and systems that are available (your own in the practice, in the PCO, outside in a training venue).
- Training that can be obtained (to match your needs).
- Training that could take place (in the practice, other practice(s), college or university, other sites such as industry, distance learning, other local or distant venue).
- How it could be done (individual or group; tutor-led or cascade learning).

By 6 months: review current performance.
- Are your skills being utilised in the best way?
- Do the building, equipment and working practices meet the specifications for the tasks you are required to perform now and those that you anticipate doing in the immediate future?

By 7 months: identify solutions and associated learning needs.
- Arrange the necessary training.
- Make a business plan for any associated equipment needs.
- Arrange cover for yourself and any other staff who are involved to provide protected time for learning.
- Clarify who does what and when.
- Negotiate changes necessary at practice meeting(s).

By 12 months: make the changes.
- Implement the new procedures.
- Obtain feedback from other staff as to the impact of changes that you make.
- Resolve any difficulties.
- Identify any gaps in the provision.

Expected outcomes: increase in uptake of smoking cessation assistance; decrease in number of smokers; maintenance of smoking cessation behaviour; fewer exacerbations of respiratory illness in ex-smokers, lower rates of cardiovascular events and other smoking-related illness. More referrals for helping patients with other addictive behaviours such as alcohol or eating disorders, as the skills for identifying problems and readiness for change are similar to those for smoking cessation.

How does your personal development plan tie in with other strategic plans? (for example the business or development plan, the local Health Improvement and Modernisation Plan, the Primary Care Investment Plan)

Make sure that your objectives mesh with others. They may have a priority for the prevention of smoking-related illness or the development of shared protocols for the management of smoking cessation between primary, intermediate and secondary care, into which you can feed your personal development plan.

What additional resources will you require to execute your plan and from where do you hope to obtain them?

Your entitlement to reimbursement of course fees, etc. will depend on your contract and on the priority value that the practice, workplace, trust or PCO puts on your development plan to meet their own needs.

Any additional equipment, alterations to the use of the building, working practices, will have to be decided on the same basis.

How will you evaluate your learning plan?

Look at the methods you used to identify your learning needs – how does it all fit? Can you repeat a measure that you adopted to establish your learning needs to determine how much you have learnt or the extent to which your performance has improved?

How will you know when you have achieved your objectives?

You will be able to carry out the tasks you have set yourself, or will have implemented the changes specified in your objectives list; most of these can be audited to measure change.

How will you disseminate the learning from your plan to the rest of the team and to patients? How will you sustain your new-found knowledge or skills?

You might let everyone, especially patients and the wider public, know in a practice newsletter. Let the staff know what has been achieved, or what is now available, at team meetings.

Pass on your skills to other people in the team as required. Keep using your skills to provide information or better working practices. You could run an in-house training session to teach others in the practice team how to do one or more of the new procedures you have mastered, e.g. search and audit.

How will you handle new learning requirements as they crop up?

Keep a record as they arise to consider later or add them in if essential at this stage.

Check whether the topic you have chosen to learn is a priority and the way in which you plan to learn about it is appropriate

> **Your topic**: *management of smoking cessation.*

How have you identified your learning need(s)?

(*a*) PCO or trust requirement	☒	(*e*) Appraisal need	☐
(*b*) Part of the business plan	☒	(*f*) New to post	☐
(*c*) Legal mandatory requirement	☐	(*g*) Individual decision	☒
(*d*) Job requirement	☐	(*h*) Patient feedback	☐
		(*i*) Other	☐

Have you discussed or planned your learning needs with anyone else?

Yes ☒   No ☐   If so, who? *Other staff; clinical tutor and clinical governance lead*

What are your learning need(s) and/or objective(s) in terms of the following?

Knowledge. What new information do you hope to gain to help you do this?

To learn how to implement strategies for the management of smoking cessation.

Skills. What should you be able to do differently as a result of undertaking this learning in your development plan?

Identify best working practices; correct poor working practices; identify risky situations; identify at risk groups and implement prevention.

Behaviour/professional practice. How will this impact on the way in which you then subsequently do things?

Regular reviews of services; regular reviews of standards of care for target groups.

Details and date of desired development activity:

Within three months: collect sufficient information. Within six months: start to implement changes to working practices and management of target groups with information and interactive sessions with those patients and staff and with the wider public.

Details of any previous training and/or experience you have in this area/ dates:

Piecemeal self-instruction without structure or specific objectives.

What is your current performance in this area compared with the requirements of your job?

Need significant development ☒   Need some development in ☐
in this area   this area

Satisfactory in this area   ☐   Do well in this area   ☐

What is the level of job relevance that this area has to your role and responsibilities?

Has no relevance to job   ☐   Has some relevance   ☐

Relevant to job   ☐   Very relevant   ☒

Essential to job   ☐

Describe how the proposed education/training is relevant to your job:

Integral part of my work in the practice team.

Do you need additional support in identifying a suitable development activity?

Yes   ☒   No   ☐

What do you need?

To know when and where relevant sessions of training are being held. Help in accessing the basic information. Help with setting up staff, patient and public sessions. Help in developing services.

Describe the differences or improvements for you, your practice, PCO or employing NHS trust as a result of undertaking this activity:

I will be able to evaluate the working practices, standards of equipment and premises, standards of prevention and management, monitor performance and assess progress towards targets set by the team and PCO.

Assess the priority of your proposed educational/training activity:

Urgent ☐   High ☒   Medium ☐   Low ☐

Describe how the proposed activity will meet your learning needs rather than any other type of course or training on the topic:

A multi-disciplinary approach is needed as the subject encompasses so many disciplines and areas of clinical and non-clinical work.

If you had a free choice would you want to learn this? *Yes*/No

If No, why not? (please circle all that apply)

Waste of time
I have already done it
It is not relevant to my work or career goals
Other

If Yes, what reasons are most important to you? (put them in rank order)

To improve my performance	1
To increase my knowledge	2
To get promotion	
I am just interested in it	
To be better than my colleagues	
To do a more interesting job	
To enable me to be more confident	3
Because it will help me	4

Record of your learning about the management of smoking cessation

You would write in the topic, date, length of time spent, etc. for each learning activity

	Activity 1 – knowledge of best practice in the provision of smoking cessation services	*Activity 2 – increase knowledge and skills about nicotine replacement therapies (NRT)*	*Activity 3 – setting up public involvement*	*Activity 4 – setting up a search and audits for monitoring best practice*
In-house formal learning	Arrange for an innovator from another district to talk to the practice team and other invited professionals	Arrange for an expert to talk about NRTs to the practice team; draw up a list of provision and indications	Health promotion to provide a speaker on how public involvement can be achieved	Set up learning sessions in the practice with the people who have skills in this area
External courses	Attend a conference on the various ways smoking cessation services are provided in other districts, and how to facilitate, change and identify readiness for change	Attend a clinic where NRTs are prescribed to learn more and gain new skills	Attend a course that includes presentations on public involvement in other districts	
Informal and personal	Read articles about what others have done; discuss how these ideas can be implemented in the workplace and PCO	Discussion with practice team and PCO about how provision and targeting could be improved; practise and disseminate what has been learned	Talking to others who have done this before; involving other members of the practice team including the health visitors, district nurses and school nurses; involving schools; community resources	Informal sessions with team members; practising the extraction of necessary data; ensuring that data is entered in a consistent way
Qualifications and/or experience gained	Attendance certificate; increased confidence in facilitating changes of behaviour	Attendance certificate; increased knowledge about NRT	Experience in public participation and liaison with non-medical and paramedical sources of help	Speed and accuracy of data production and report writing

Template for your personal development plan

What topic have you chosen?

Who chose it?

Why is the topic a priority?

(i) A personal and professional priority?

(ii) A practice or workplace priority?

(iii) A district priority?

(iv) A national priority?

Who will be included in your personal development plan?
(Anyone other than you? Doctors, employed staff, attached staff, others from outside the workplace, patients?)

What baseline information will you collect and how?

How will you identify your learning needs?
(How will you obtain this information and who will do it? Self-completion check-lists, discussion, appraisal, audit, patient feedback?)

What are the learning needs of the practice or workplace and how do they match your needs?

Is there any patient or public input to your personal development plan?

Aims of your personal development plan arising from the preliminary data-gathering exercise

How might you integrate the 14 components of clinical governance into your personal development plan focusing on the topic of . . . . ?

Establishing a learning culture:

Managing resources and services:

Establishing a research and development culture:

Reliable and accurate data:

Evidence-based practice and policy:

Confidentiality:

Health gain:

Coherent team:

Audit and evaluation:

Meaningful involvement of patients and the public:

Health promotion:

Risk management:

Accountability and performance:

Core requirements:

Action learning plan
(Include timetabled action and expected outcomes)

How does your personal development plan tie in with other strategic plans?
(e.g. the practice's or workplace's business or development plan, the local Health Improvement and Modernisation Plan, the Primary Care Investment Plan?)

What additional resources will you require to execute your plan and from where do you hope to obtain them?
(Will you have to pay any course fees? Will you be able to organise any protected time for learning in working hours?)

How will you evaluate your learning plan?

How will you know when you have achieved your objectives?
(How will you measure success?)

How will you disseminate the learning from your plan to the rest of the team and to patients? How will you sustain your new-found knowledge or skills?

How will you handle new learning requirements as they crop up?

Check whether the topic you have chosen to learn is a priority and the way in which you plan to learn about it is appropriate.

Your topic:

How have you identified your learning need(s)?

(a) PCO/trust requirement ☐ (e) Appraisal need ☐

(b) Part of the business plan ☐ (f) New to post ☐

(c) Legal mandatory requirement ☐ (g) Individual decision ☐

(d) Job requirement ☐ (h) Patient feedback ☐

(i) Other ☐

Have you discussed or planned your learning needs with anyone else?

Yes ☐ No ☐ If yes, who?

. . . .

What are your learning need(s) and/or objective(s) in terms of the following?

Knowledge. What new information do you hope to gain to help you to do this?

. . . .

Skills. What should you be able to do differently as a result of undertaking this learning in your development plan?

. . . .

Behaviour/professional practice. How will this impact on the way in which you then subsequently do things?

. . . .

Details and date of desired development activity:

. . . .

Details of any previous training and/or experience you have in this area/dates:

. . . .

What is your current performance in this area compared with the requirements of your job?

Need significant development ☐   Need some development ☐
in this area   in this area

Satisfactory in this area ☐   Do well in this area ☐

What is the level of job relevance that this area has to your role and responsibilities?

Has no relevance to job ☐   Has some relevance ☐

Relevant to job ☐   Very relevant ☐

Essential to job ☐

Describe how the proposed education/training is relevant to your job:

. . . .

Do you need additional support in identifying a suitable development activity?

                        Yes ☐   No ☐

What do you need?

. . . .

Describe the differences or improvements for you, your workplace, PCO or employing NHS trust as a result of undertaking this activity:

. . . .

Assess the priority of your proposed educational/training activity:

   Urgent ☐   High ☐   Medium ☐   Low ☐

Describe how the proposed activity will meet your learning needs rather than any other type of course or training on the topic:

. . . .

If you had a free choice, would you want to learn this?   Yes/No

If No, why not? (please circle all that apply)

Waste of time
I have already done it
It is not relevant to my work or career goals
Other

If Yes, what reasons are most important to you? (put them in rank order)

To improve my performance
To increase my knowledge
To get promotion
I am just interested in it
To be better than my colleagues
To do a more interesting job
To enable me to be more confident
Because it will help me

Record of your learning activities

Write in the topic, date, time spent, type of learning, etc., for each learning activity

	Activity 1	Activity 2	Activity 3	Activity 4
In-house formal learning				
External courses				
Informal and personal				
Qualifications and/or experience gained				

References

1 Chambers R, Wakley G and Iqbal Z (2001) *Cardiovascular Disease Matters in Primary Care*. Radcliffe Medical Press, Oxford.

2 Wakley G, Chambers R and Field S (2000) *Continuing Professional Development in Primary Care: making it happen.* Radcliffe Medical Press, Oxford.

3 *Guidelines in Practice*. Medendium Group Publishing Ltd. www.eguidelines.co.uk .

4 Chambers R (2000) *Involving Patients and the Public*. Radcliffe Medical Press, Oxford.

5 Chambers R and Wakley G (2000) *Making Clinical Governance Work for You*. Radcliffe Medical Press, Oxford.

CHAPTER 10

Draw up and apply your practice or workplace personal and professional development plan

The practice or workplace personal and professional development plan (PPDP) should cater for everyone who works in the practice. Clinical governance principles will balance the development needs of the population, the practice or department, the primary care organisation (PCO) or trust *and* your individual personal development plan (PDP).

You might want to start by identifying your own learning needs, combining them with those of other people and then checking them against the practice or departmental business plan. You could start from the other direction, and develop a practice- or department-based personal and professional development plan from your business plan and then identify your individual learning needs within that. Whichever direction you start from, you must ensure that you integrate your individual needs with those of your practice and the needs and directives of the NHS.

Your learning plan should complement the professional development of other individuals and that of the practice or department. If you are working on a project that involves change for other people as well as yourself, it is better to work together towards a common goal and co-ordinate multi-professional learning across traditional boundaries. Multi-professional learning does not mean sitting together all learning the same information; rather that you all learn together and individually as appropriate to your roles and responsibilities. All the team members will then understand and respect each other's contributions to provide co-ordinated patient-centred care.

If you work in a number of different roles or posts, gaps and duplication of activities should be avoided. After reflection on the boundaries between your roles, you may be able to focus your learning so that meeting your needs in one role benefits another.

Make your learning plan flexible. You may want to add something in later if circumstances suddenly change or an additional need becomes apparent – perhaps as the result of a complaint, a new drug being released onto the market or hearing something new at a meeting.

Remember to include all those staff who work for the practice or department, however few their hours – you cannot manage without them or they would not be there! Long-term locums (greater than six months, say), assistants, retained doctors and salaried or staff grade doctors should all be included in the practice or workplace plan.

Time is one of the resources that must be considered when drawing up your action plan. Adequate resources must be in place for your learning needs, and protected time must be built in to your plan.

Worked example of a practice or workplace personal and professional development plan: providing guidelines for pharmacological interventions for smoking cessation in a trust or PCO

Who chose the topic?

The use of pharmacological interventions has been shown to be haphazard and inconsistent after a preliminary assessment from the prescribing data and annual reports. The district or PCO is undertaking a review of the provision of pharmacological interventions after advice from the pharmaceutical adviser and the guidance from NICE.

Why is the topic a priority?

(i) A practice or professional priority? Good risk management is an essential part of care at a clinical level for individuals. Risk management is also important from an organisational perspective in identifying those at risk, preventing unwanted adverse effects and providing best management of need. So investing time and effort in improving the way in which pharmacological interventions are used results in gains for individual patients.

(ii) A district priority? Several other districts have already set up guidelines or protocols for the use of pharmacological interventions in smoking cessation, e.g. the programme used in Dorset[1] in the South

of England. They have local initiatives to co-ordinate the management of those who require smoking cessation services and they provide smoking cessation specialist advice by GPs and nurses with special interest and skills.

(iii) A national priority? The cost of the effects of failing to assist people with stopping smoking is high. Effective prevention is cost-effective to the NHS, through avoiding premature death and reducing morbidity, and minimising the effects of poor health on physical and psychosocial functioning. NICE has advised that pharmacological interventions should be available nationally for everyone living in England.

Who will be included in your practice or workplace personal and professional development plan?

You might include the following:

- patients who want to stop smoking
- health promotion advisers
- community pharmacists
- GPs
- practice nurses
- school nurses
- health visitors
- district nurses
- practice managers
- reception staff
- representatives from education and social services
- representatives from community and secondary care
- representatives from the wider public.

Who will collect the baseline information and how?

A computer operator could do an electronic search in practices or workplaces to identify those who have, or should have, received pharmacological interventions, and the risk factors that might prevent their use, if appropriately coded. It will be a laborious process setting up an at-risk register of people who should not receive pharmacological interventions from discharge letters from hospital, paper records, repeat prescriptions, recall, etc.

A needs assessment of your area might be used by the PCO or trust to establish what proportion of people will require pharmacological inter-ventions and where these will best be based.

Where are you now (baseline)?

- Establish how many people smoke and how many may be considering stopping. Set up criteria for identifying high priority groups you might tackle to start with (e.g. those with cardiovascular disease, diabetes, antenatal patients, young women on oral contraceptives, parents of young children).
- List the risk factors, giving relative or absolute contraindications to pharmacological interventions; try to ensure that they will be flagged up automatically in computer prescribing systems if you aim to prescribe for patients who have risk factors.
- Compare any local practice guidelines for pharmacological interventions with a guideline cited in the literature as 'best practice', or a district protocol or guideline from elsewhere. If you have not got practice guidelines write them or modify ones that are already available.[2,3]
- Assess the quantity and quality of literature available for patients and their partners.
- Review the extent of education or training the clinical staff have received about pharmacological interventions.
- Undertake an analysis of the strengths, weaknesses, opportunities and threats (SWOT) of your PCO or trust in writing and implementing guidelines and protocols.

What information will you obtain about individual learning wishes and needs?

You might review practice protocols and baseline information with as many staff as possible at discussion groups and find out whether they feel competent as individuals to carry out their roles and responsibilities, or want to realign their duties. They might comment on how well others are fulfilling their responsibilities and suggest improvements to the systems or procedures that have educational and resource consequences – training sessions, new equipment, and especially the effects on other parts of the practice organisation of introducing new provisions or ways of working.

Significant event audits, such as of a patient who had a fit after receiving buproprion, or another who is continuing to use nicotine chewing gum frequently, after trying it to give up smoking, might help to clarify any problems.

What are the learning needs of the practice or workplace and how do they match individual staff needs?

Responding to the queries from the PCO or trust about the provision of pharmacological interventions might reveal inadequacies of information about what services are being provided, how they are utilised or what they achieve. This should create the opportunity to review how individuals contribute to the overall service provided – include the employed and attached staff as well as individuals such as the local community pharmacist or the local youth worker. Once you are sure of everyone's roles and responsibilities and your vision for the care you intend to provide, you can re-assess individuals' learning needs in a co-ordinated plan to match the service you will provide.

Compare your own figures for numbers of people who would require pharmacological interventions with those you would expect in a population of your size and demographic make-up. Conclude whether you need to be more proactive in identifying those in need and those who should not receive pharmacological interventions. Address any lack of knowledge or skills, uncaring or disillusioned attitudes in staff, or inadequate systems.

Compare prescribing patterns between the GPs in your area with other areas. Look for differences and inconsistencies that may indicate learning needs.

A patient's complaint may reveal learning needs for individuals or the practice organisation, e.g. from a patient who was told to buy her nicotine replacement therapy when she might have been prescribed it without being charged.

Compare available practice guidelines for the management of smoking cessation with other recommended guidelines to reveal the staff's learning needs.

A practice managers' group may intend to visit other areas to find out how others manage their services for the provision of a smoking cessation service. This focus might justify additional time spent on practice or clinic visiting.

Is there any patient or public input to your practice or workplace development plan?

Ask the patient who made a complaint or comment to help you to devise better systems for the practice, or to write an account of their experiences that can be used for a training session.

You might ask the pharmacist or an expert who has set up a service elsewhere to run training sessions for implementing the guidelines – in particular, dealing with educating and informing patients better, teaching patients about risks and the side-effects of treatment.

An open forum on smoking cessation and pharmacological interventions can be held for all those staff who will be involved to provide an opportunity for everyone to mix and exchange ideas; informal conversations during the evening should reveal learning needs and ideas for improvements.

Aims of the practice or workplace personal and professional development plan arising from the preliminary data-gathering exercise

After gathering baseline data and undertaking a preliminary learning needs assessment you might design a practice personal and professional development plan with the grand aims:

- of developing suitable guidelines on effective smoking cessation and pharmacological interventions to pilot in the practice or workplace

and

- of developing a learning programme for all members of the practice or workplace team, attached staff and individuals to enable them to implement the guidelines on effective smoking cessation and pharmacological interventions

or

- you might concentrate on enabling particular key individuals, e.g. a GP or practice nurse and a specific receptionist from the practice or workplace team with lead responsibility, for implementing the guidelines on effective smoking cessation and pharmacological interventions. They could then cascade their learning in-house to others in the practice or workplace team.

And then:

- roll out the programme across the PCO or trust to provide good standards and cost-effective management of smoking cessation throughout the area.

How might you integrate the 14 components of clinical governance into your practice personal and professional development plan focusing on developing guidelines on effective smoking cessation and pharmacological interventions?

Establishing a learning culture: a multidisciplinary team might update their learning about effective smoking cessation and pharmacological interventions.

Managing resources and services: promote close working relationships and teamwork. Provide new services to fill the gaps and reduce duplication of effort. Advertise services that are available to all the population in the area of one PCO or trust.

Establishing a research and development culture: encourage team members to critically appraise published papers which describe new findings of pharmacological interventions for smoking cessation, to check whether the results described are applicable to the PCO or trust's population.

Reliable and accurate data: keep good records to enable evaluation of the service provided and to establish how it can be monitored and improved.

Evidence-based practice and policy: the guidelines on effective smoking cessation and pharmacological interventions should be based on the best evidence available for the population and on local circumstances.

Confidentiality: there should be water-tight systems in place to prevent any information about a patient accessing smoking cessation services being released without their consent. Any issues of confidentiality should be clarified before information about individuals is passed to others. Data should be collected and anonymised before leaving a practice or department.

Health gain: increased rates of smoking cessation improve health and well being and reduce the health-related costs to the individual and society.

Coherent team: all the practice team should understand each others' roles and responsibilities in providing care.

Audit and evaluation: a significant event audit of, for example, a person with risk factors and on pharmacotherapy having a fit, or someone not being prescribed suitable nicotine replacement therapy, should indicate areas where further training is required, or where practice services and teamwork should be improved.

Meaningful involvement of patients and the public: you might hold a public session in the surgery, or elsewhere, to demonstrate strategies for meeting smoking cessation needs. An assessment questionnaire for identifying needs might define areas that are not being met. A focus group of patients with smoking cessation needs might reveal shortcomings in staff knowledge and attitudes, or malfunctioning practice systems, or a lack of appropriate services.

Health promotion: target patients who smoke with advice about their lifestyles, not through negative messages but as part of increasing their ability to enjoy life in a healthy way.

Risk management: identifying and controlling risks is part of the purpose for providing guidelines on effective smoking cessation and pharmacological interventions.

Accountability and performance: demonstrate that the advice and treatment staff are providing to people receiving smoking cessation services is in line with best practice.

Core requirements: staff should be competent and trained for their roles and responsibilities; think about skill mix and other appropriately trained professionals, e.g. health advisors or counsellors, ex-smokers with suitable skills, to supplement the expensive skills of specialised staff.

Action learning plan

Agree who is involved/setting: people as set out previously – specify names, posts, timetabled action, start date.

By 3 months: preliminary data-gathering and collation of baseline of providers of smoking cessation services.
- Guidelines or protocols are collected and one is prepared for local conditions.
- Numbers of staff identified; map expertise available; list other sources of expertise.
- Information is collated about characteristics of those recorded as having needs for smoking cessation and pharmacological interventions – age groups, ethnic origins, etc.
- Define any relevant local and national priorities; and any additional associated resources for which you might apply.
- Hold staff and patient discussion to report problems that limit or prevent access by those with unmet needs and their views and suggestions.

By 4 months: review current performance.
- Start to review the implementation of the guidelines.
- Clinical lead (e.g. GP, nurse) reviews extent of knowledge, skills and attitudes of practice or departmental team in respect of how well the guidelines are followed.
- Audit actual performance versus pre-agreed criteria, e.g. with respect to how well the guidelines are followed and what difficulties arise.
- Compare performance with any or several of the 14 components of clinical governance, for example, health promotion would be relevant.

By 6 months: identify solutions and associated training needs.
- Revise the guidelines. Address any identified gaps in care or knowledge having undertaken searches for other evidence-based guidelines. Agree roles and responsibilities as a team for delivering care and services according to protocols or guidelines.
- Plan the training for all or selected relevant personnel from practices or departments on important aspects of the guidelines.

By 12 months: make changes.
- Evaluate clinicians' adherence to guidelines – as shown by repeat audits and patient feedback.
- Modify guidelines in line with recent evidence and new medications available.
- Re-assess educational needs in the PCO or trust and start the roll out to the PCO or trust.

Expected outcomes: standardisation and better adherence to best practice for smoking cessation and pharmacological interventions; better quit rates of smoking cessation; improved public health; reductions in rates of smoking-related illnesses, morbidity and death.

How does your practice personal and professional development plan tie in with other strategic plans?

The business plan for the practice or department and the PCO's or trust's investment plan might both prioritise achieving a more effective smoking cessation programme. The practice personal and professional development plan that focuses on providing a generic guideline for the PCO or trust would complement those strategic plans.

What additional resources will you require to execute your plan and from where do you hope to obtain them?

The practice or department might pay the course fees of any member of staff undertaking training that fulfils a priority need of the practice or department.

You may be able to justify an application for additional resources to your PCO or trust with your preliminary learning and health needs assessments, tapping into the district or national strategic priorities. You should point out that this expenditure would be balanced by savings from the increased rate of smoking cessation.

If a member of staff is undertaking the training on behalf of the practice or workplace you should try to arrange that the training is undertaken in paid time. Any learning cascaded to other members of the practice or workplace team as part of the personal and professional development plan should also be undertaken in paid time and during working hours whenever possible.

How will you evaluate your practice or workplace personal and professional development plan?

You should be able to pick out methods of evaluation from the range of methods you use for assessing learning needs. The most appropriate methods will depend on what specific aims you set for your development plan. If your main aim is to standardise the prescription of pharmacological interventions across the PCO or trust, then you might start with an assessment of the level of education and training needed, meet these needs and then monitor the prescriptions and any adverse effects.

If your aim was to improve the levels and appropriateness of education and information for people with previously unmet needs for help with smoking cessation, you might want to ask the patients themselves – by a simple test of knowledge, focus group discussion of experiences, monitoring changes in patient behaviour, etc.

The administrative and clinical leads for implementing the guidelines for the PCO or trust (e.g. a practice manager and GP or practice nurse) might plan the evaluation together and delegate the collection of data to a clerical assistant.

How will you know when you have achieved your objectives?

Usually this will be by comparing outcomes of your programme with baseline data. This might be achieved by comparing the use of pharmacological interventions before and after the implementation of the guidelines. It might be also determined by looking at patients' compliance with recommended practice, or the lifestyle changes they have achieved.

How will you disseminate the learning from your plan to the rest of the team and patients? How will staff sustain their new-found knowledge and skills?

You might write about what has been learnt in a newsletter. Let all the staff know at practice meetings what progress has been made. You might want to describe your success at a PCO meeting or apply for an award for best practice from one of the national medical or health service news sheets, before rolling out the new service to the rest of the PCO or trust.

Pass on your skills and knowledge to others as required and review your guidelines at set intervals to incorporate new information.

How will you handle new learning requirements as they crop up?

The administrative lead might run audits at intervals and feed the results back to practice or departmental meetings. This might take place mid-way through the time period of the development plan when there is time to revise the activities.

Record of practice team learning about the development of guidelines for pharmacological interventions for smoking cessation

You would add the date, length of time spent, etc. for each learning activity

	Activity 1 – revise existing guidelines and protocols	Activity 2 – update staff education	Activity 3 – piloting the generic guideline	Activity 4 – involving patients and the public
In-house formal learning	Team discussion around roles and responsibilities of various members to revise and modify guidelines and any necessary patient group directions	Lead people run in-house sessions on best practice on the place of pharmacological interventions in smoking cessation advice	The guidelines are piloted with monitoring of who is prescribed nicotine replacement or buproprion to determine any deviations or risks not included. Results fed back at staff meeting	Health education advisor runs a session on change and awareness of readiness to change for staff. Then facilitates an open session with staff and patients on a Saturday morning and a Wednesday evening
External courses	Lead clinician attends continuing education course on pharmacological interventions			Lead clinician attends a course on management of behaviour change
Informal and personal	Lead clinician and administrator search for examples of best practice on the practice computer.[4,5] Lead administrator rings round other practices and clinics to ask for examples of protocols and guidelines	A folder of up-to-date information on smoking cessation and pharmacological interventions is made available on the practice intranet system and in a loose-leaf folder in the common room	Discussion between staff improves the use of the guidelines and reinforces the learning previously acquired	Staff promote knowledge of smoking cessation interventions during patient encounters. Several staff use their change management knowledge to tackle personal needs
Qualifications and/or experience gained	Clinical lead receives accreditation that can be put in the learning portfolio. Both leads record their search activity	Reflective learning recording	Recording of use of guidelines and personal adherence levels or difficulties	Certificate of attendance at course, reflective learning from patient management and personal experience

Template for your practice or workplace personal and professional development plan

What topic have you chosen?

Who chose it?

Why is the topic a priority?
(i) A practice or professional priority?

(ii) A district priority?

(iii) A national priority?

Who will be included in your practice or workplace personal and professional development plan?
(GPs, nurses, employed staff, attached staff, others from outside the practice or workplace, patients?)

Who will collect the baseline information and how?

How will you identify your learning needs?
(How will you obtain this information and who will do it? Self-completion check-lists, discussion, appraisal, audit, patient feedback?)

What are the learning needs of the practice or workplace and how do they match individual staff needs?

Is there any patient or public input to your practice or workplace development plan?

Aims of your practice or workplace personal and professional development plan arising from the preliminary data-gathering exercise

**How might you integrate the 14 components of clinical govern-
ance into your practice personal and professional development
plan focusing on the topic of . . . . ?**

Establishing a learning culture:

Managing resources and services:

Establishing a research and development culture:

Reliable and accurate data:

Evidence-based practice and policy:

Confidentiality:

Health gain:

Coherent team:

Audit and evaluation:

Meaningful involvement of patients and the public:

Health promotion:

Risk management:

Accountability and performance:

Core requirements:

Action learning plan
(Include timetabled action and expected outcomes)

How does your practice or workplace personal and professional development plan tie in with other strategic plans?
(e.g. the practice's business or development plan, the local Health Improvement and Modernisation Plan, the Primary Care Investment Plan, the trust's development plan?)

What additional resources will you require to execute your plan and from where do you hope to obtain them?
(Will staff have to pay any course fees? Will they be able to organise any protected time for learning in working hours?)

How will you evaluate your practice or workplace personal and professional learning plan?

How will you know when you have achieved your objectives?
(How will you measure success?)

How will you disseminate the learning from your plan to the rest of the team and patients? How will you sustain your new-found knowledge and skills?

How will you handle new learning requirements as they crop up?

Record of your learning

Write in the topic, date, time spent, etc., for each learning activity

	Activity 1	Activity 2	Activity 3	Activity 4
In-house formal learning				
External courses				
Informal and personal				
Qualifications and/or experience gained				

References

1 Russ P (2001) *Nurse-led Smoking Cessation Group Proves Successful.* www.eguidelines.co.uk .

2 West R, McNeill A and Raw M (2000) Smoking cessation guidelines for professionals: an update. *Thorax.* **55**: 537–40.

3 British Heart Foundation (2001) *Stopping Smoking.* British Heart Foundation, London. Also www.bhf.org.uk .

4 Raw M, West R and McNeill A (2001) Smoking cessation guidelines updated to clarify strategies. *Guidelines in Practice.* Medendium Group Publishing Ltd. www.eguidelines.co.uk .

5 www.quit.org.uk gives useful links.

The stages of change

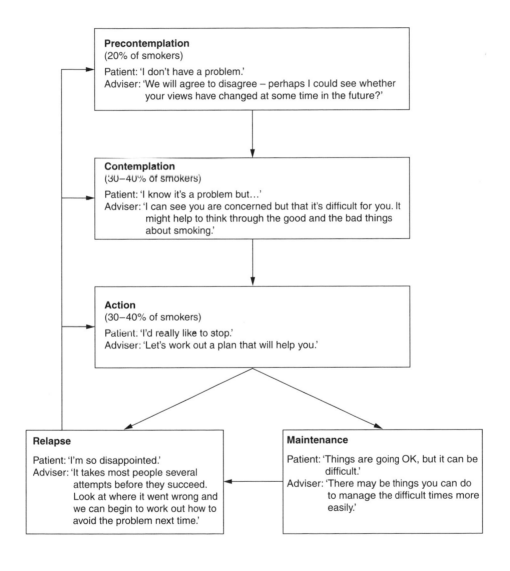

Precontemplation
(20% of smokers)

Patient: 'I don't have a problem.'
Adviser: 'We will agree to disagree – perhaps I could see whether your views have changed at some time in the future?'

Contemplation
(30–40% of smokers)

Patient: 'I know it's a problem but…'
Adviser: 'I can see you are concerned but that it's difficult for you. It might help to think through the good and the bad things about smoking.'

Action
(30–40% of smokers)

Patient: 'I'd really like to stop.'
Adviser: 'Let's work out a plan that will help you.'

Relapse

Patient: 'I'm so disappointed.'
Adviser: 'It takes most people several attempts before they succeed. Look at where it went wrong and we can begin to work out how to avoid the problem next time.'

Maintenance

Patient: 'Things are going OK, but it can be difficult.'
Adviser: 'There may be things you can do to manage the difficult times more easily.'

Carbon monoxide monitoring

A carbon monoxide breath monitor is a useful and relatively cheap tool for smoking cessation work. It shows the amount of carbon monoxide in parts per million (ppm CO) in the breath, and is an indirect, non-invasive measure of blood carboxyhaemoglobin levels (% COHb).

In a 'typical' puff of cigarette smoke there is about 5% carbon monoxide by volume. The half-life of carbon monoxide inhaled in this way is about 5 to 6 hours. Usually after a maximum period of 48 hours the ex-smoker would show the same level as a non-smoker living in the same environment.

For smoking cessation purposes:

- levels of 0–10 are characteristic of a non-smoker
- levels of 11–20 are characteristic of a light smoker
- levels of 21–100 are characteristic of a heavy smoker.

Carbon monoxide monitoring is predominantly a motivational tool to give the smoker visible proof of the damaging carbon monoxide levels and to help by charting their progress during the programme.

Prescribing nicotine replacement therapy

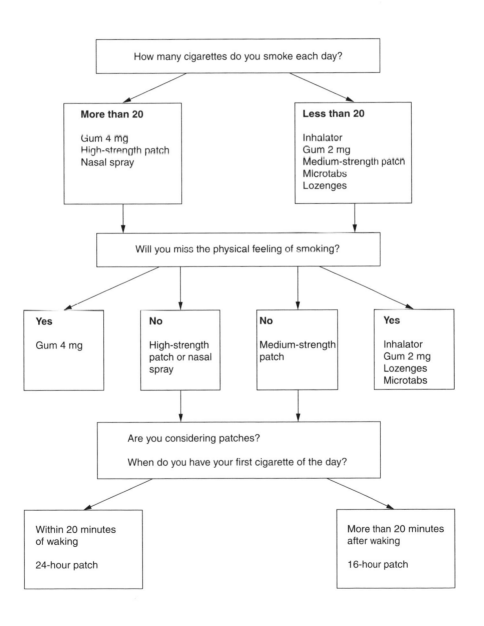

How many cigarettes do you smoke each day?

More than 20

Gum 4 mg
High-strength patch
Nasal spray

Less than 20

Inhalator
Gum 2 mg
Medium-strength patch
Microtabs
Lozenges

Will you miss the physical feeling of smoking?

Yes

Gum 4 mg

No

High-strength patch or nasal spray

No

Medium-strength patch

Yes

Inhalator
Gum 2 mg
Lozenges
Microtabs

Are you considering patches?

When do you have your first cigarette of the day?

Within 20 minutes of waking

24-hour patch

More than 20 minutes after waking

16-hour patch

A practice protocol

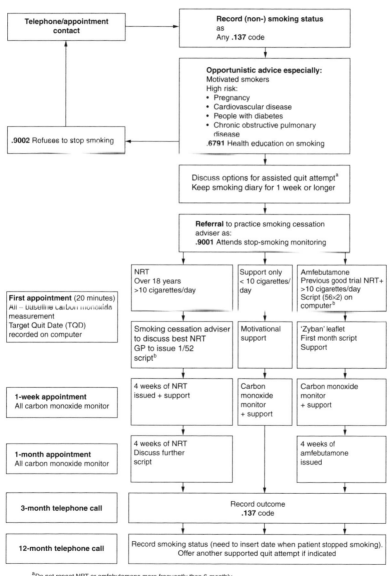

Telephone/appointment contact	**Record (non-) smoking status** as Any **.137** code

Opportunistic advice especially:
Motivated smokers
High risk:
- Pregnancy
- Cardiovascular disease
- People with diabetes
- Chronic obstructive pulmonary disease
.6791 Health education on smoking

.9002 Refuses to stop smoking

Discuss options for assisted quit attempt[a]
Keep smoking diary for 1 week or longer

Referral to practice smoking cessation adviser as:
.9001 Attends stop-smoking monitoring

	NRT	Support only	Amfebutamone
	Over 18 years >10 cigarettes/day	< 10 cigarettes/ day	Previous good trial NRT+ >10 cigarettes/day Script (56×2) on computer[b]
First appointment (20 minutes) All – baseline carbon monoxide measurement Target Quit Date (TQD) recorded on computer	Smoking cessation adviser to discuss best NRT GP to issue 1/52 script[b]	Motivational support	'Zyban' leaflet First month script Support
1-week appointment All carbon monoxide monitor	4 weeks of NRT issued + support	Carbon monoxide monitor + support	Carbon monoxide monitor + support
1-month appointment All carbon monoxide monitor	4 weeks of NRT Discuss further script		4 weeks of amfebutamone issued
3-month telephone call	Record outcome **.137** code		
12-month telephone call	Record smoking status (need to insert date when patient stopped smoking). Offer another supported quit attempt if indicated		

[a] Do not repeat NRT or amfebutamone more frequently than 6-monthly.
[b] Nurse smoking adviser may recommend amfebutamone, but it is the GP's responsibility to check the prescription.

Draft workplace smoking policy (ASH)

Smoking policy for (*name of organisation*) _____

Effective from (*date*) _____

Introduction

Passive smoking – breathing other people's tobacco smoke – has now been shown to cause lung cancer and heart disease in non-smokers, as well as many other illnesses and minor conditions.

Section 2(2)(e) of the Health and Safety at Work Act 1974 places a duty on employers to provide a working environment for employees that is: '. . . safe, without risks to health, and adequate as regards facilities and arrangements for their welfare at work.'

The employer acknowledges that breathing other people's tobacco smoke is both a public health hazard and a welfare issue. Therefore the following policy has been adopted concerning smoking in (*name of organisation*) _____

General principles

This smoking policy seeks to guarantee non-smokers the right to work in air free of tobacco smoke, whilst also taking account of the needs of those who smoke.

All premises will be designated smoke-free from (*date*) _____
with a limited number of clearly marked separate smoking rooms. Smoking will only be allowed in the separate rooms, which may not be used for any other purpose. Smoking while on duty will only be allowed during official break periods.

Common areas

Smoking is not permitted in the following areas.

- Lifts
- Corridors
- Stairways
- Restaurant/canteen
- Rest rooms
- Meeting rooms
- Toilets
- Reception areas
- Entrances
- Car parks
- Other areas (*specify as necessary*) _____

Work areas

Smoking is not permitted in any work area. This applies to all offices and work areas, whether occupied by one person, or shared by two or more. Anyone who wishes to smoke must do so during official break periods and only in the designated smoking rooms.

Smoking rooms

Designated smoking rooms are provided at (*locations*) _____

The employer will ensure that the smoking rooms are kept clean and are properly ventilated. Contaminated air from the smoking rooms will not enter the general air circulating in the rest of the building.

Vehicles

Smoking is not permitted in official vehicles. (*what to do about company cars which are taken home*)

The policy of no smoking will apply to the car park.

Unions/Health and Safety representative

This policy has been devised in full consultation with all of those employees who are concerned with health and safety in this workplace. It enjoys the support of the relevant representatives.

Informing staff of the policy

The employer has informed staff 90 days in advance and will provide all members of staff with a copy of this policy upon their request.

Visitors and temporary staff

Visitors and temporary staff are expected to abide by the terms of this policy. The following arrangements have been made for informing them of its existence.

* Adequate signage
* Receptionist/person greeting them will explain the policy.

Recruitment procedures

Job advertisements, job descriptions and interviews will include reference to this policy. On their appointment, all new staff members will be given a copy of this policy.

Help for those who smoke

This policy recognises that passive smoking adversely affects employees' health. It is not concerned with *whether* anyone smokes, but with *where* they smoke, and the effect that this has on non-smoking colleagues. However, it is recognised that the smoking policy will impact on smokers' working lives. In an effort to help individuals adjust to this change, the following help is being provided.

* Up to five hours off to attend any course that will help smokers to quit.
* Smoking cessation support provided by (*specify*).

Enforcement of the policy

Breaches of this policy will be subject to the normal disciplinary procedures.

Implementation, monitoring and review

Responsibility for implementing and monitoring this policy rests with senior managers. Twelve weeks' notice will be given of the introduction of this policy.

Monitoring this policy will be carried out at three, six and twelve months following its implementation.

A formal review of the policy will be conducted after eighteen months. Trade unions and health and safety representatives will be consulted over the results of the monitoring and review.

Changes to the policy

Twelve weeks' notice will be given of any changes made to the policy. Trade unions and health and safety representatives will be consulted in good time about any proposed changes.

Resources

QUIT

Victory House
170 Tottenham Court Road
London W1T 7NR
Quitline: 0800 00 22 00
Website: www.quit.org.uk

A UK charity that helps smokers to quit. Counsellors offer confidential help and advice about every aspect of quitting. They offer a variety of more tailored support which includes minority ethnic communities, pregnancy, young people and a Dads' quitline.

Don't Give Up Giving Up

Website: www.givingupsmoking.co.uk

An NHS website, with content authored by the Health Development Agency, which provides information on how to give up smoking

GASP

93 Cromwell Road
Bristol BS6 5EX
Tel/Fax: +44 (0)117 942 5185
Email: gasp@gasp.org.uk
Website: http://www.gasp.org.uk
Provides smoking cessation posters, literature, leaflets and presentations.

ASH (Action on Smoking and Health)

102 Clifton Street
London EC2A 4HW
Tel: +44 (0)20 7739 5902
Fax: +44 (0)20 7613 0531

Email: action.smoking.health@dial.pipex.com
Website: http://www.ash.org.uk

STOP! Magazine

Website: www.stopmagazine.co.uk

Features celebrity interviews and success stories with up-to-date information on treatments and techniques for smokers who want to quit.

Bedfont Scientific Ltd

Website: www.bedfont.com

Manufacturers of 'smokerlyzer' carbon monoxide breath-measuring devices for use in smoking cessation settings.

Index

Page numbers in *italics* refer to figures and tables.